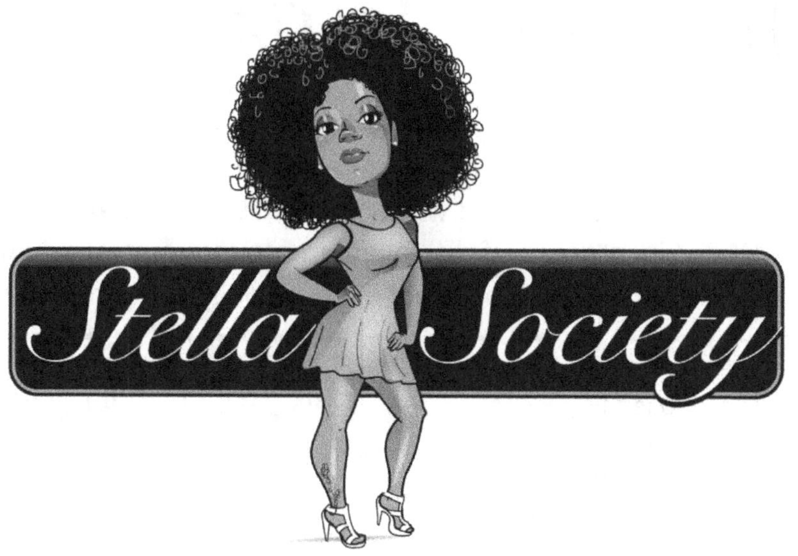

Thank you for participating in the Stella Project 2.0, a 40 day fitness confidence and nutrition challenge.
If you purchased this journal and you are not a member of the Stella Project, no worries. You can find us at stellasocietyacademy dot com, or just use it on your own 40 day fitness journey.

Always consult a physician before beginning an exercise program.

How to use your journal

Journaling has many benefits especially when tracking progress. Recording your thoughts before training can help you better understand why a workout did or didn't go too well. Recalling the times you eat and what can help you combat unnecessary cravings. Journaling also increases self-discipline, improves your mood and boost comprehension. Please use this journal to aid in your goals through your 40 days.

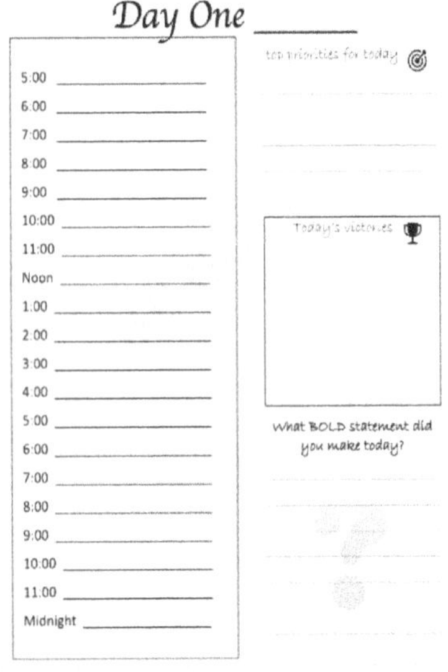

Use this page to record your daily schedule, meals, training, meetings, etc. Make sure you put the date. List your top priorities hat must be completed that day. Record your victories, like drinking all your water and reflect on the daily bestellatude

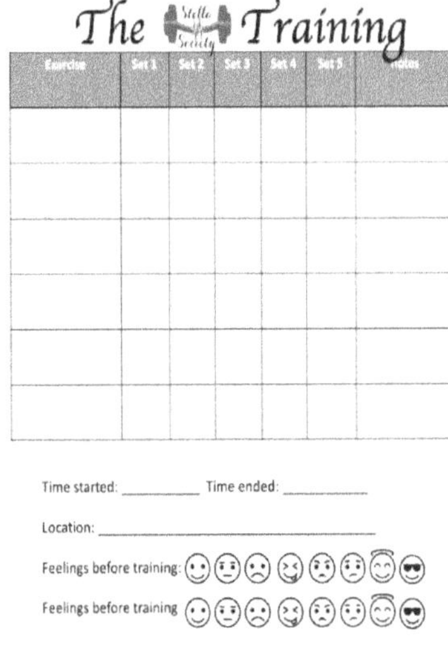

Use this page to record your training sessions. Write them down ahead of time and watch the video in case you have questions. Put the time your started and completed the training as well as how you felt before and after. Leave a note as to why you felt a certain before the training. This could effect how it went.

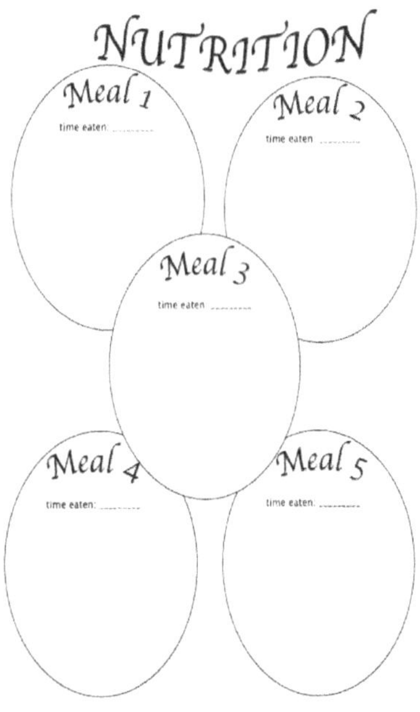

Use this page to record your meals and the time you ate them. This is important especially when tracking your progress. Try to eat your meals at the same time each day. Get your machine on a schedule so it knows how to operate its fuel.

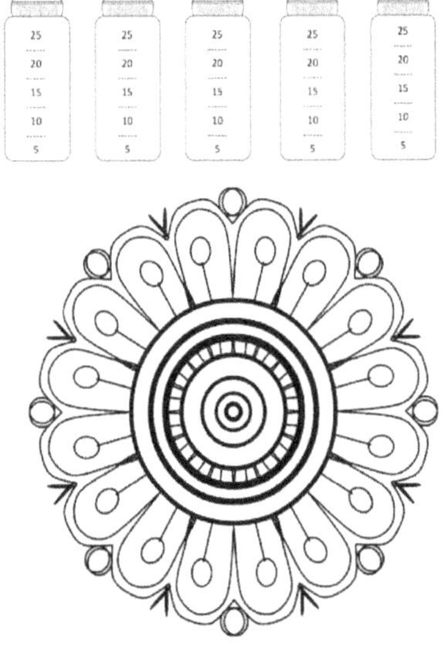

Use this page to record your water intake. Color the bottles as you complete each one. Also each hydration page has a mandala graphic to color. Coloring is a form of meditation. Choose to color this instead of reaching for something to snack on that's not you're your meal plan.

R.O.S.E.S GOAL

Rationale – why are you participating in this 40 day challenge?

____

____

Objective – what do you look to accomplish during the 40 days? What is the end game, goal?

____

____

Strategy – how will you go about completing your objective? What actions will you take.

____

____

Evaluation – how and when will you evaluate you progress? Will you use inches, weight, look, or clothes?

____

____

Schedule – create a schedule for the next 40 days. Include anything that will get in the way of your goal and find a work around.

____

____

Measurements

DATE: __________

Weight: ______

Neck ______

Shoulders ______

Chest ______

Bicep / upper arm left _______ right ______

Forearm left _______ right ______

Waist ______

Hips ______

Thighs left _______ right ______

Calf left _______ right ______

Only I Can Change My Life, No One Can Do It For Me

Day One _______

5:00 _______________	

5:00 _______________

6:00 _______________

7:00 _______________

8:00 _______________

9:00 _______________

10:00 _______________

11:00 _______________

Noon _______________

1:00 _______________

2:00 _______________

3:00 _______________

4:00 _______________

5:00 _______________

6:00 _______________

7:00 _______________

8:00 _______________

9:00 _______________

10:00 _______________

11:00 _______________

Midnight _______________

top priorities for today

____
____
____
____
____

Today's victories

What BOLD statement did you make today?

____
____
____
____
____
____
____

The Stella Society Training

Exercise	Set 1	Set 2	Set 3	Set 4	Set 5	notes

Time started: _____________ Time ended: _______________

Location: ____

Feelings before training: 🙂 😐 ☹️ 😜 😠 😟 😇 😎

Feelings after training 🙂 😐 ☹️ 😜 😠 😟 😇 😎

NUTRITION

Meal 1

time eaten: _________

Meal 2

time eaten: _________

Meal 3

time eaten: _________

Meal 4

time eaten: _________

Meal 5

time eaten: _________

Hydration

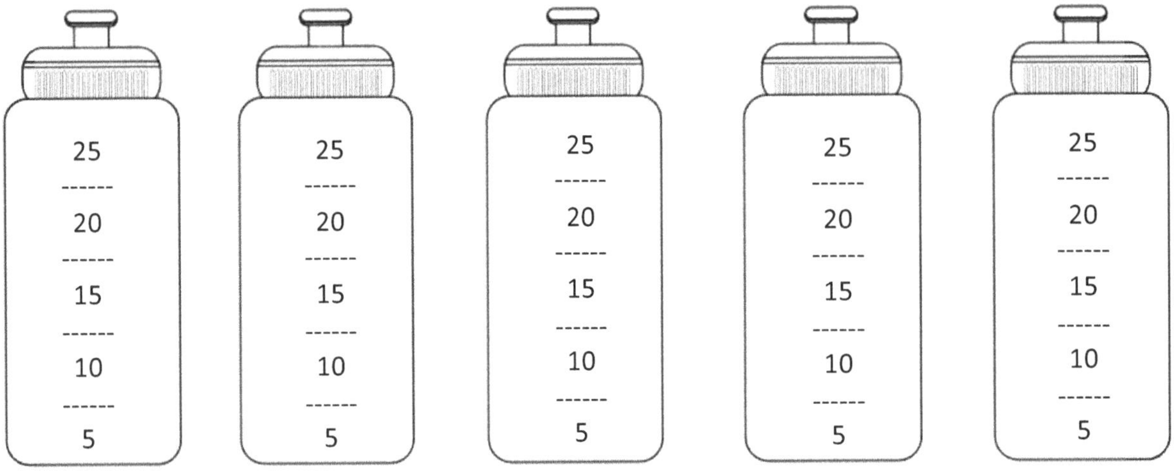

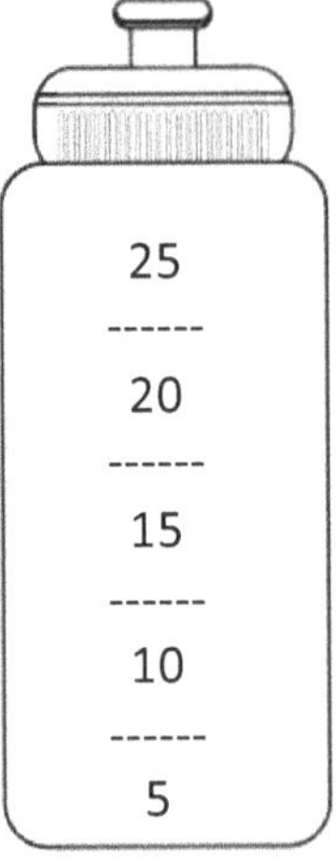

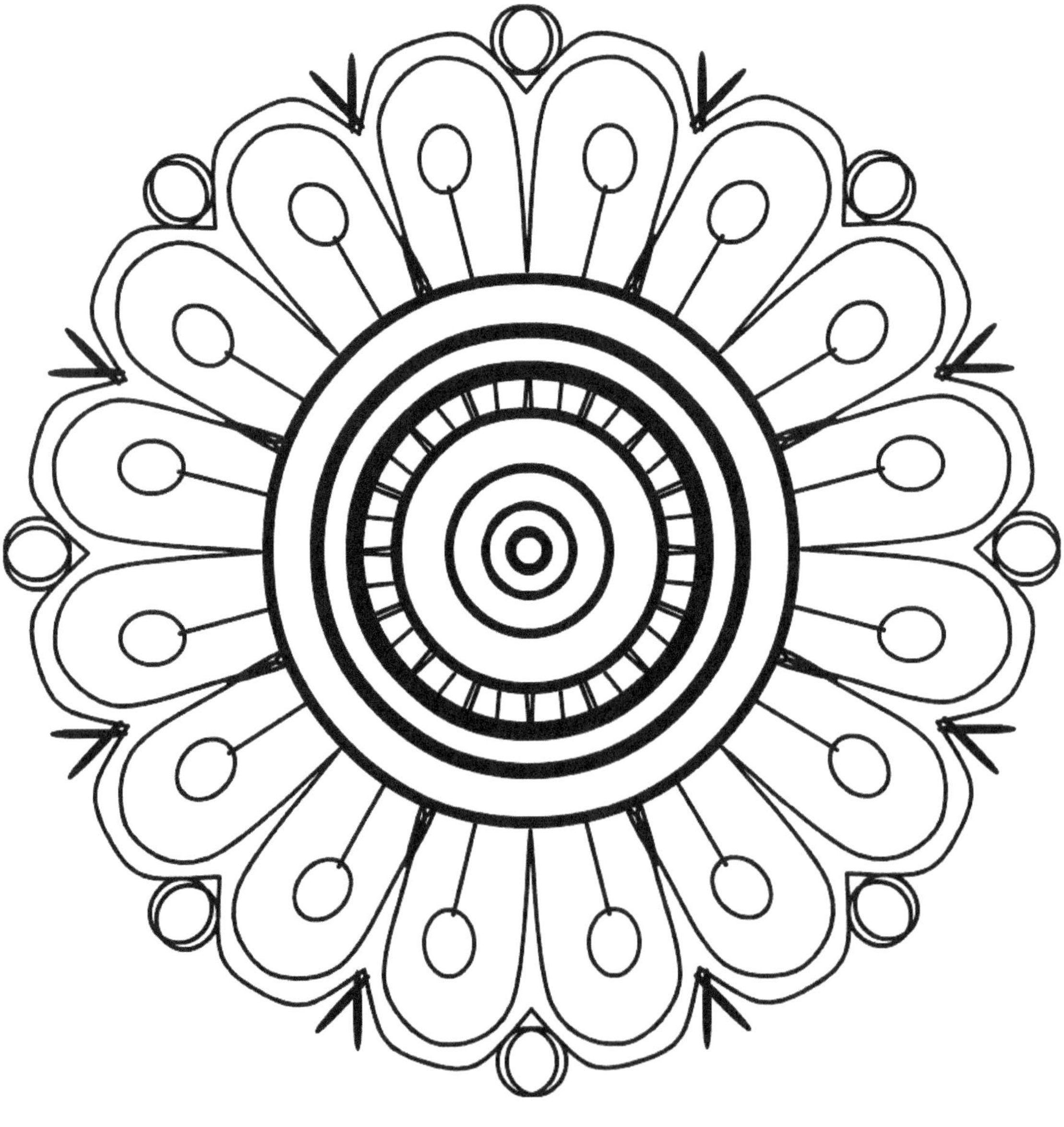

Day Two _______

5:00 _________________________	

5:00 _________________________

6:00 _________________________

7:00 _________________________

8:00 _________________________

9:00 _________________________

10:00 ________________________

11:00 ________________________

Noon _________________________

1:00 _________________________

2:00 _________________________

3:00 _________________________

4:00 _________________________

5:00 _________________________

6:00 _________________________

7:00 _________________________

8:00 _________________________

9:00 _________________________

10:00 ________________________

11:00 ________________________

Midnight ______________________

top priorities for today

____

____

____

____

____

Today's victories 🏆

What is one thing that makes you unique??

____

____

____

____

____

____

____

The *Stella Society* Training

Exercise	Set 1	Set 2	Set 3	Set 4	Set 5	notes

Time started: _____________ Time ended: _______________

Location: ____

Feelings before training:

Feelings after training

NUTRITION

Meal 1

time eaten: _________

Meal 2

time eaten: _________

Meal 3

time eaten: _________

Meal 4

time eaten: _________

Meal 5

time eaten: _________

Hydration

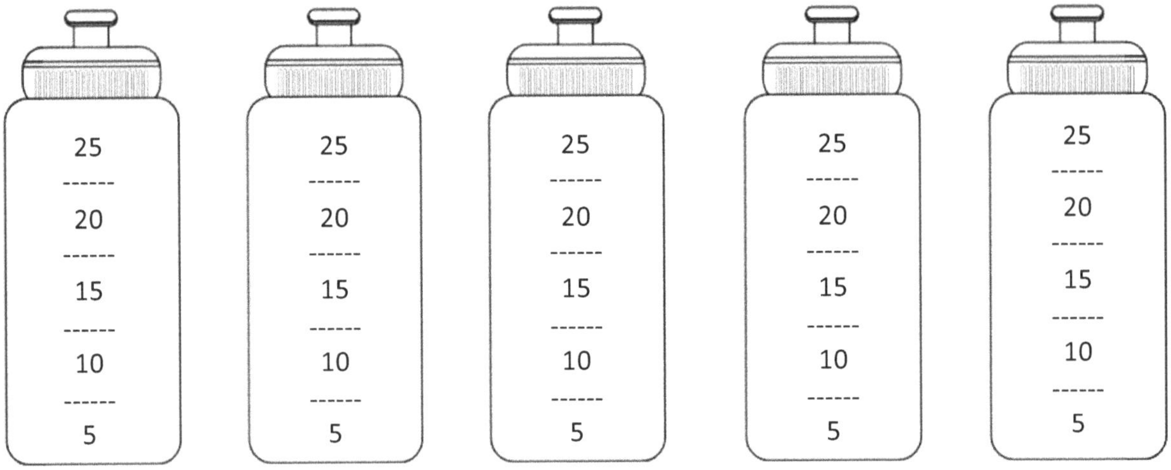

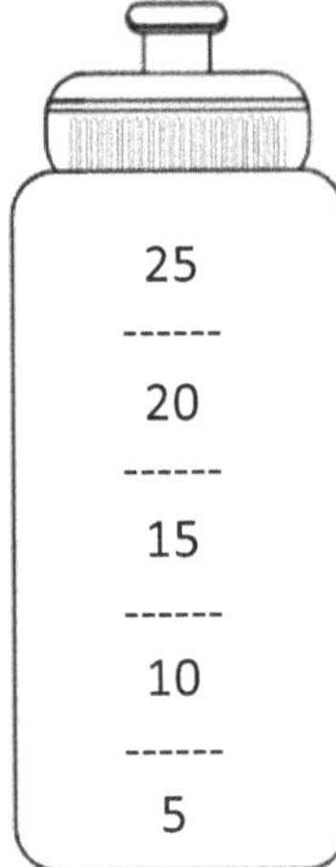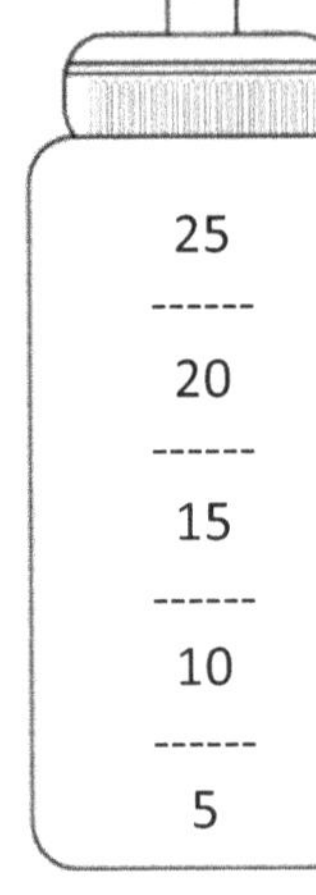

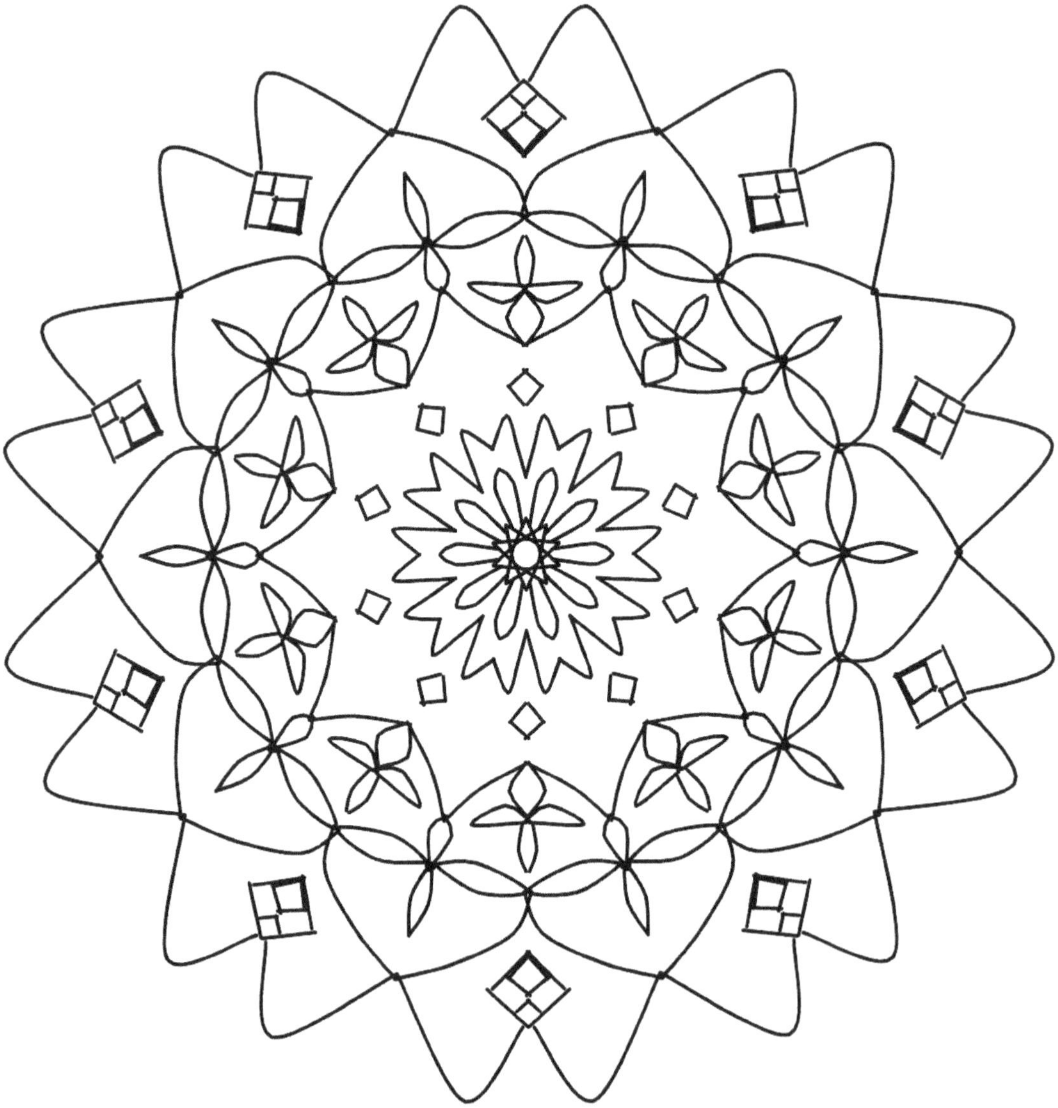

Day Three ________

5:00 ____________________	
6:00 ____________________	
7:00 ____________________	

top priorities for today

____

____

____

____

Today's victories

What makes you brave?

____

____

____

____

____

5:00 ____________________
6:00 ____________________
7:00 ____________________
8:00 ____________________
9:00 ____________________
10:00 ____________________
11:00 ____________________
Noon ____________________
1:00 ____________________
2:00 ____________________
3:00 ____________________
4:00 ____________________
5:00 ____________________
6:00 ____________________
7:00 ____________________
8:00 ____________________
9:00 ____________________
10:00 ____________________
11:00 ____________________
Midnight ____________________

The Training

Exercise	Set 1	Set 2	Set 3	Set 4	Set 5	notes

Time started: _____________ Time ended: _____________

Location: ____

Feelings before training: 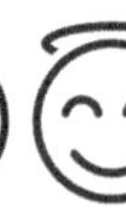

Feelings after training

NUTRITION

Meal 1

time eaten: _________

Meal 2

time eaten: _________

Meal 3

time eaten: _________

Meal 4

time eaten: _________

Meal 5

time eaten: _________

Hydration

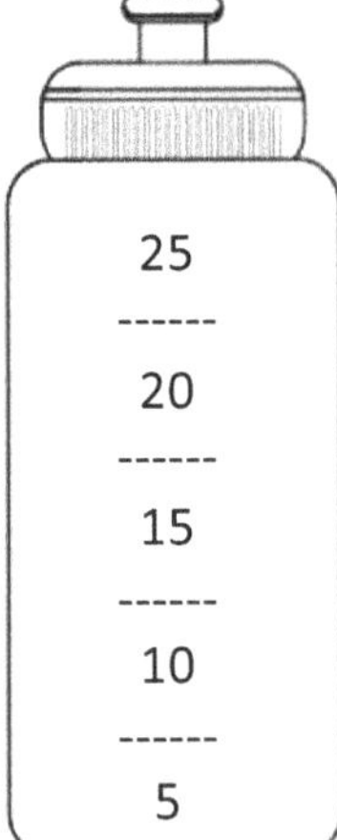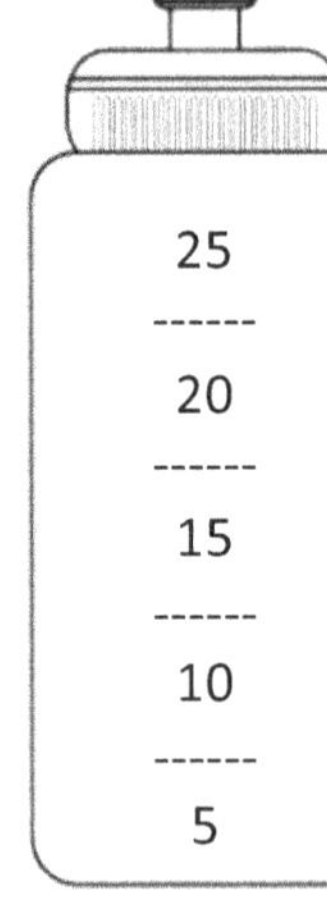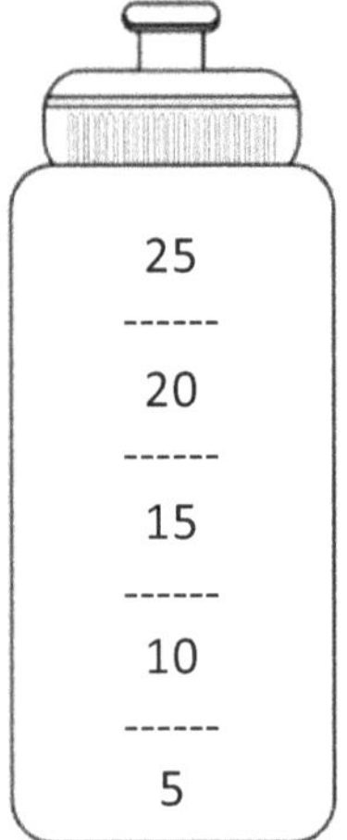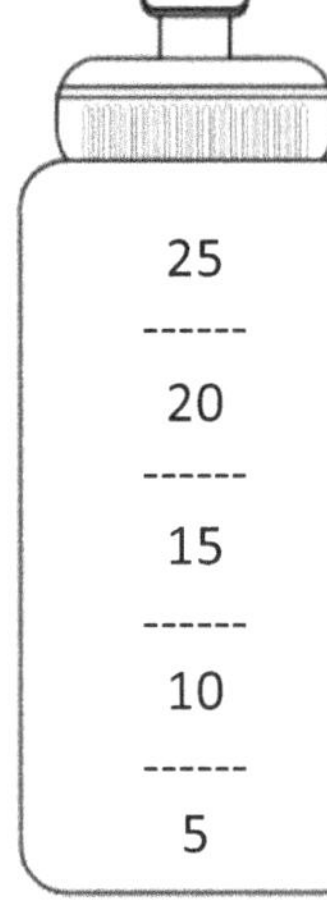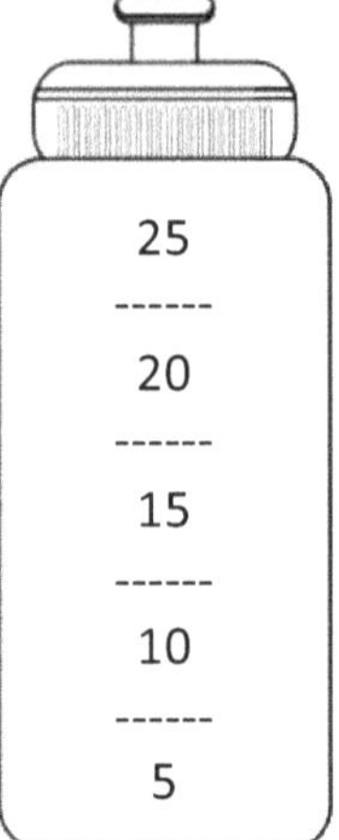

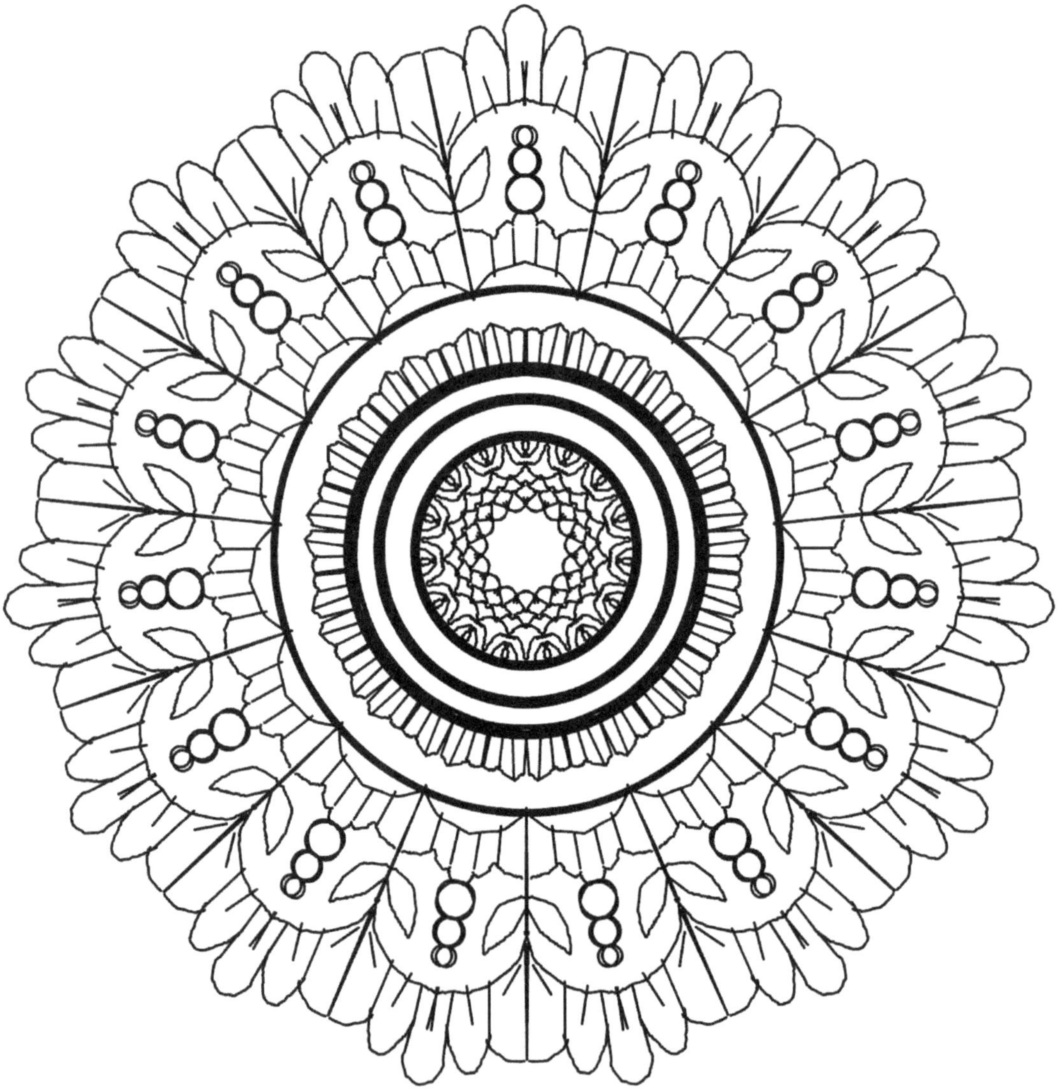

Day Four _______

5:00 ______________	

5:00 ______________
6:00 ______________
7:00 ______________
8:00 ______________
9:00 ______________
10:00 ______________
11:00 ______________
Noon ______________
1:00 ______________
2:00 ______________
3:00 ______________
4:00 ______________
5:00 ______________
6:00 ______________
7:00 ______________
8:00 ______________
9:00 ______________
10:00 ______________
11:00 ______________
Midnight ______________

top priorities for today

____
____
____
____

Today's victories

What did you commit to today that will make for a better tomorrow?

____
____
____
____
____
____

The *Stella Society* Training

Exercise	Set 1	Set 2	Set 3	Set 4	Set 5	notes

Time started: _______________   Time ended: _________________

Location: ____

Feelings before training: 😊 😐 ☹ 😜 😠 😟 😇 😎

Feelings aftertraining 😊 😐 ☹ 😜 😠 😟 😇 😎

NUTRITION

Meal 1
time eaten: _________

Meal 2
time eaten: _________

Meal 3
time eaten: _________

Meal 4
time eaten: _________

Meal 5
time eaten: _________

Hydration

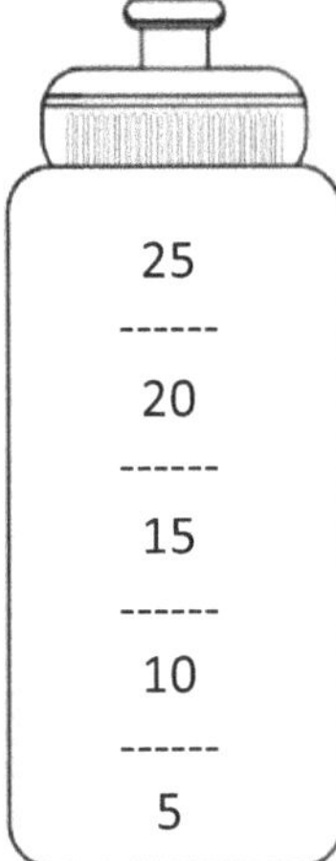 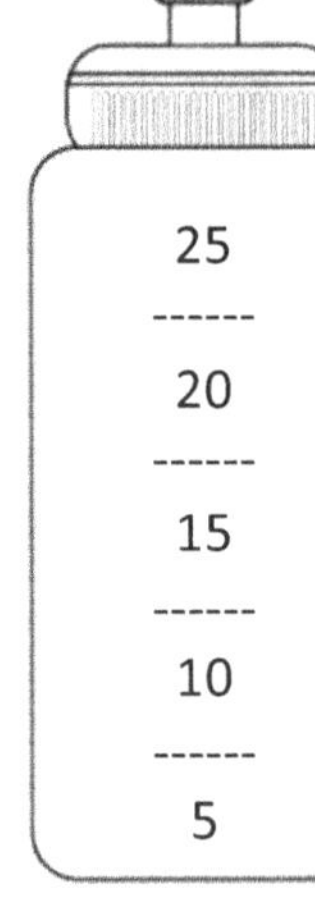 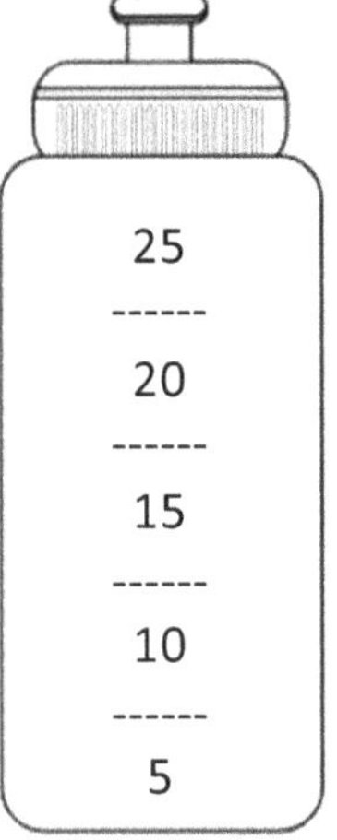 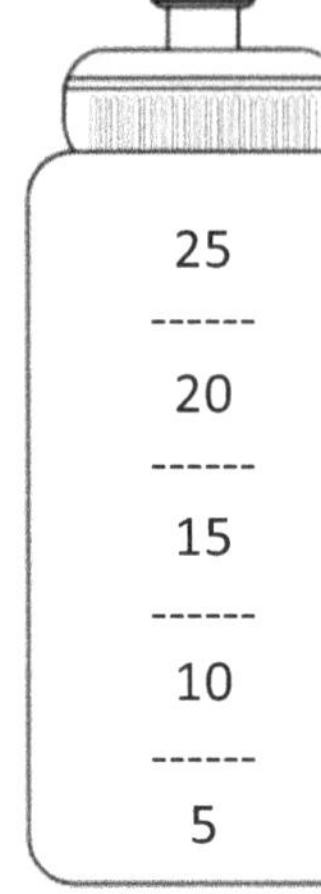 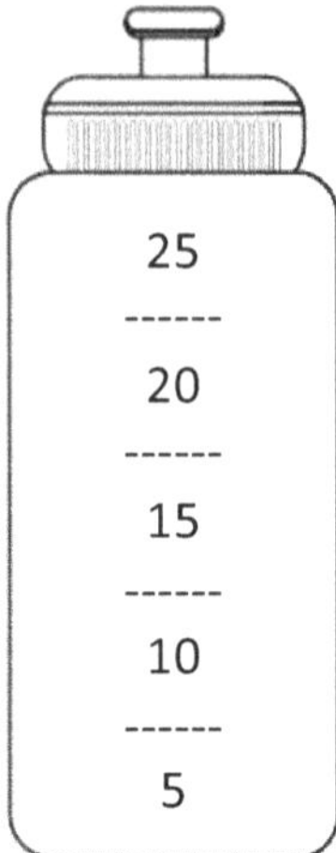

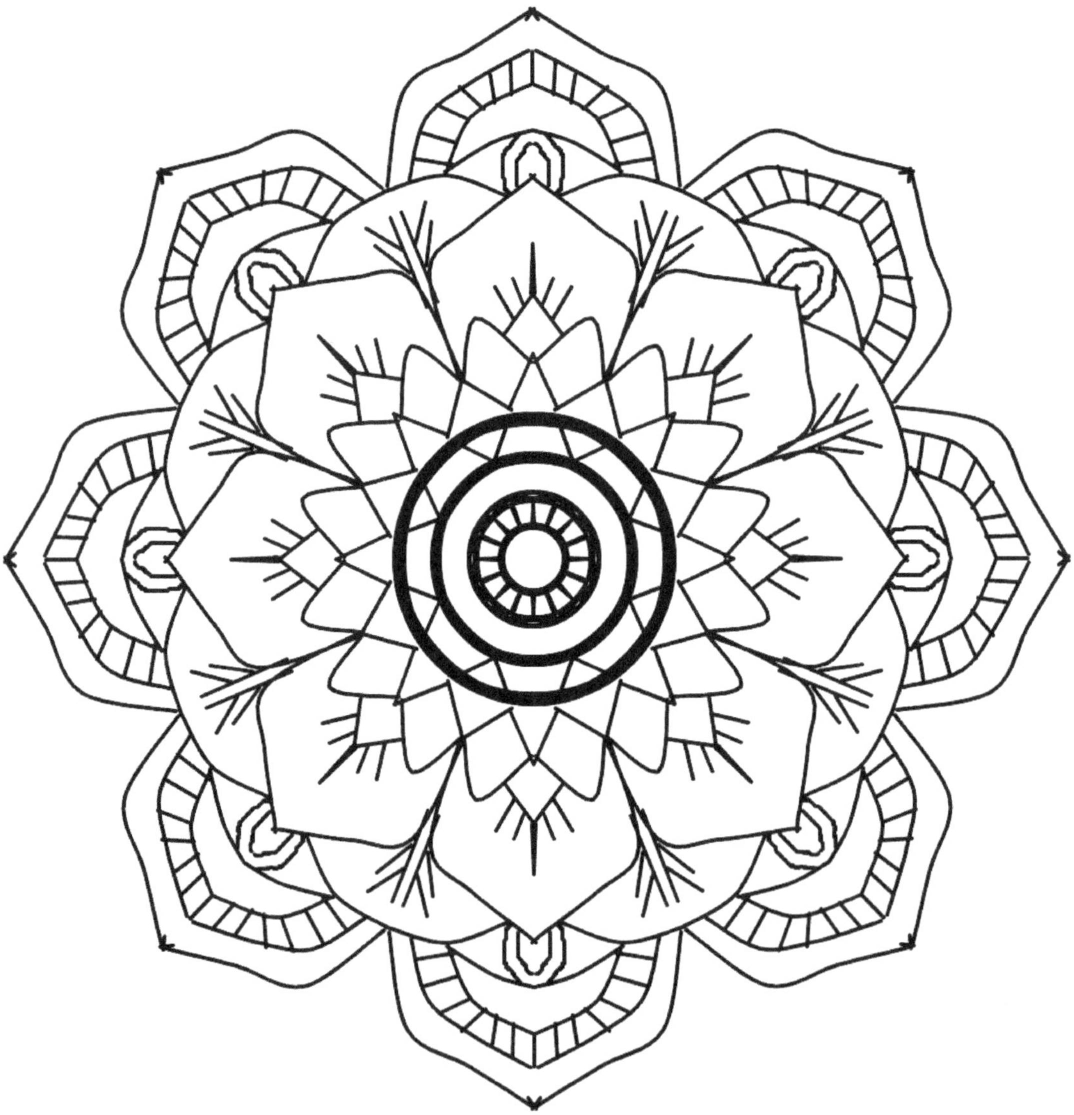

Day Five _______

<table>
<tr><td>

5:00 _______________________

6:00 _______________________

7:00 _______________________

8:00 _______________________

9:00 _______________________

10:00 ______________________

11:00 ______________________

Noon _______________________

1:00 _______________________

2:00 _______________________

3:00 _______________________

4:00 _______________________

5:00 _______________________

6:00 _______________________

7:00 _______________________

8:00 _______________________

9:00 _______________________

10:00 ______________________

11:00 ______________________

Midnight ___________________

</td><td>

top priorities for today 🎯

____

____

____

____

Today's victories 🏆

Who is the wisest person you know?
Talk to them today.

____

____

____

____

____

____

</td></tr>
</table>

The Stella Society Training

Exercise	Set 1	Set 2	Set 3	Set 4	Set 5	notes

Time started: _____________ Time ended: _______________

Location: ____

Feelings before training:

Feelings after training

NUTRITION

Meal 1

time eaten: _________

Meal 2

time eaten: _________

Meal 3

time eaten: _________

Meal 4

time eaten: _________

Meal 5

time eaten: _________

Hydration

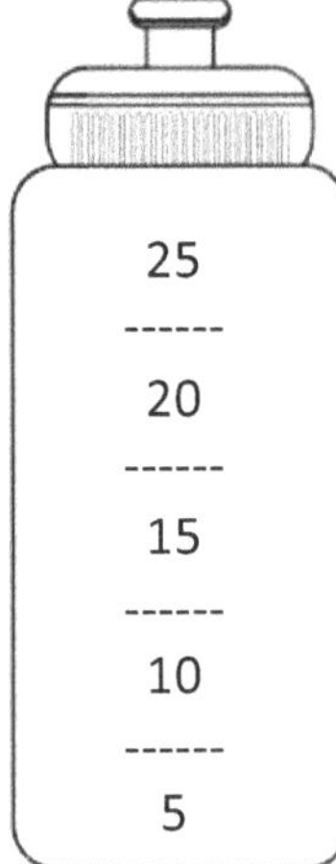

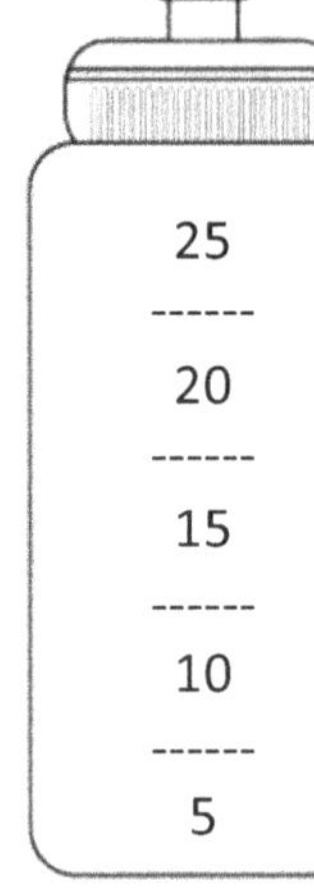

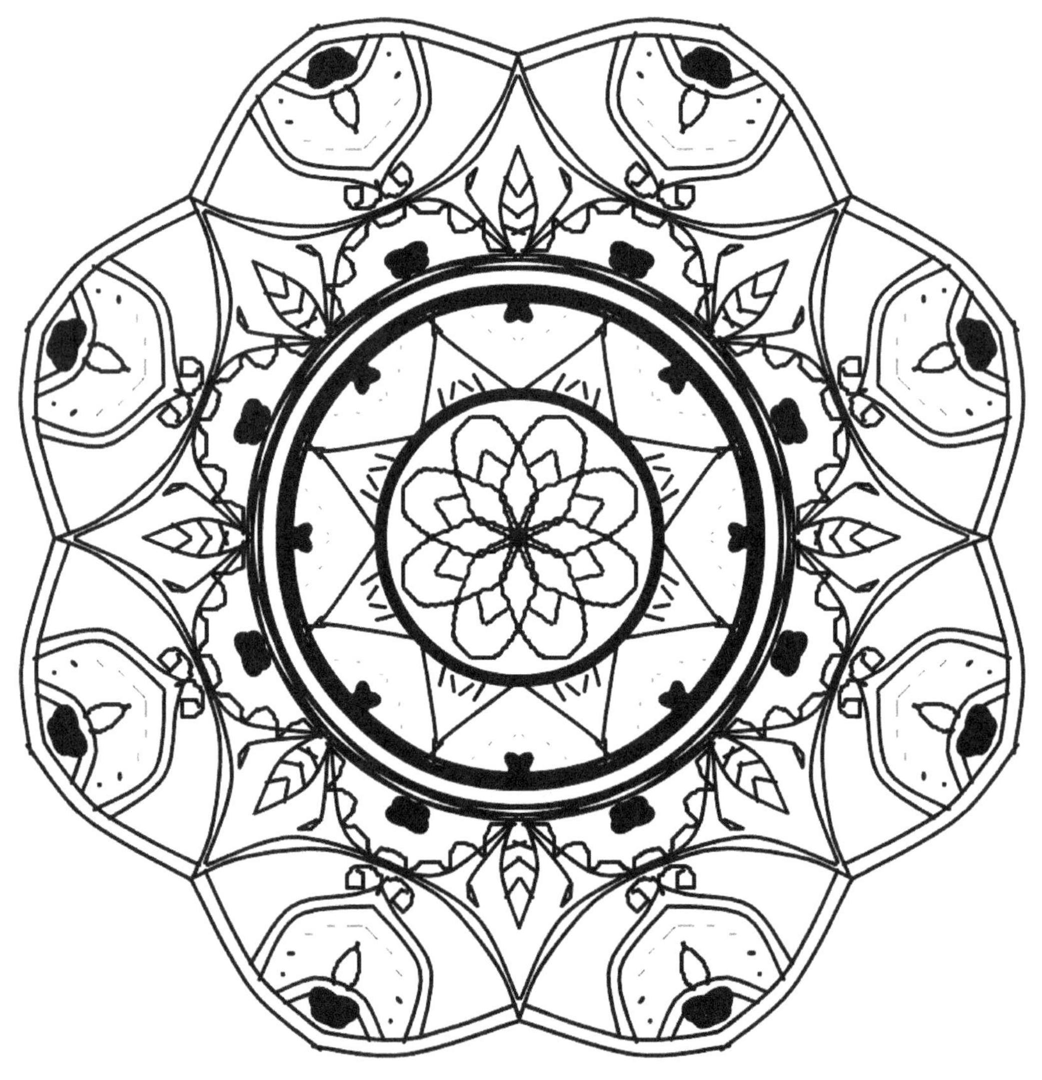

Day Six ______

5:00 _______________________

6:00 _______________________

7:00 _______________________

8:00 _______________________

9:00 _______________________

10:00 _____________________

11:00 _____________________

Noon _____________________

1:00 _______________________

2:00 _______________________

3:00 _______________________

4:00 _______________________

5:00 _______________________

6:00 _______________________

7:00 _______________________

8:00 _______________________

9:00 _______________________

10:00 _____________________

11:00 _____________________

Midnight ___________________

top priorities for today 

____

____

____

____

Today's victories 🏆

What is your biggest fear and how do you get over it?

____

____

____

____

____

____

The Stella Society Training

Exercise	Set 1	Set 2	Set 3	Set 4	Set 5	notes

Time started: _____________ Time ended: _______________

Location: ____

Feelings before training: 😊 😐 ☹️ 😜 😠 😕 😇 😎

Feelings after training 😊 😐 ☹️ 😜 😠 😕 😇 😎

NUTRITION

Meal 1

time eaten: _________

Meal 2

time eaten: _________

Meal 3

time eaten: _________

Meal 4

time eaten: _________

Meal 5

time eaten: _________

Hydration

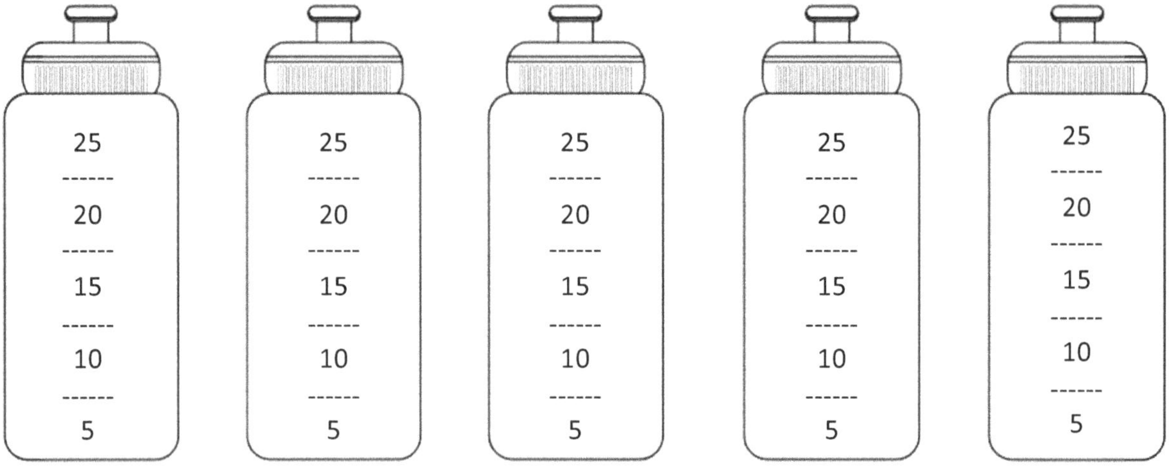

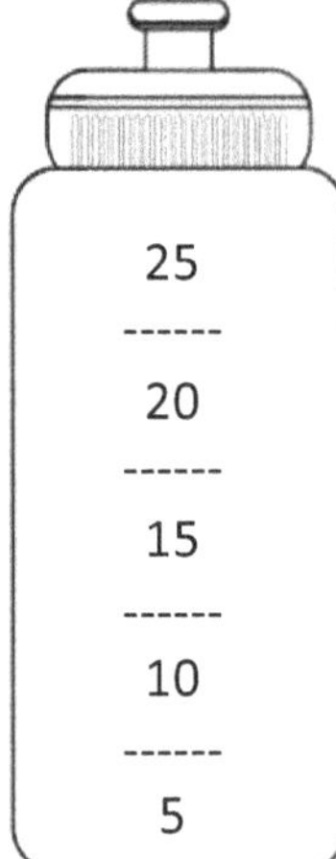
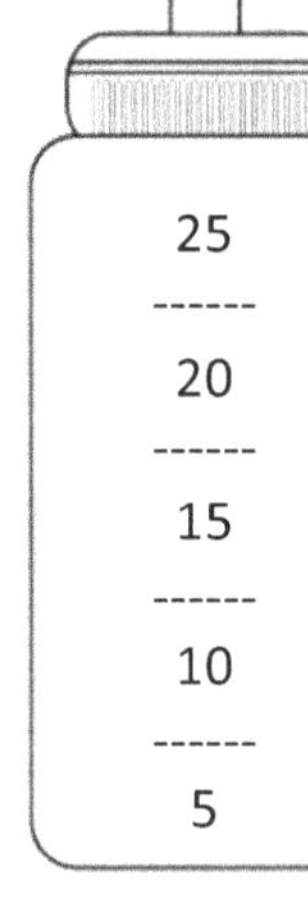
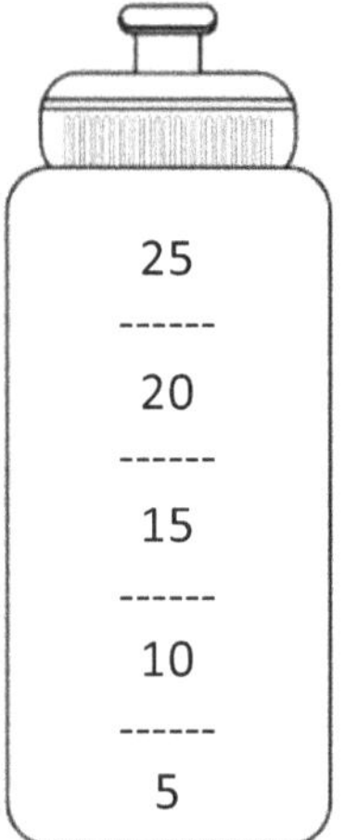

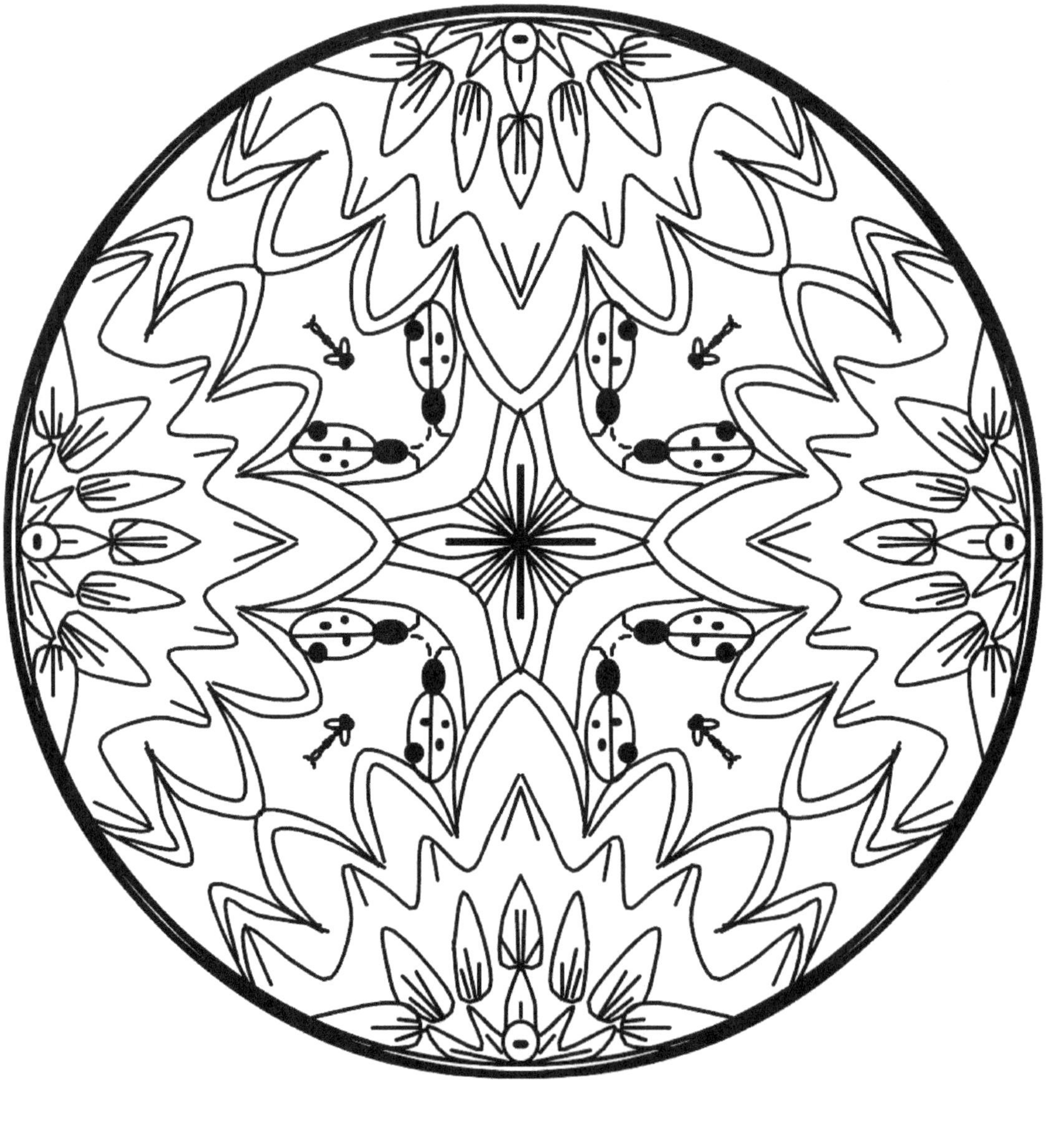

Day Seven _______

5:00 _______________	

5:00 _______________

6:00 _______________

7:00 _______________

8:00 _______________

9:00 _______________

10:00 _______________

11:00 _______________

Noon _______________

1:00 _______________

2:00 _______________

3:00 _______________

4:00 _______________

5:00 _______________

6:00 _______________

7:00 _______________

8:00 _______________

9:00 _______________

10:00 _______________

11:00 _______________

Midnight _______________

top priorities for today 🎯

____

____

____

____

Today's victories 🏆

Where does your strength
come from?

____

____

____

____

____

____

____

The *Stella Society* Training

Exercise	Set 1	Set 2	Set 3	Set 4	Set 5	notes

Time started: _______________ Time ended: _______________

Location: ____

Feelings before training: 😊 😐 ☹ 😜 😠 😕 😇 😎

Feelings after training 😊 😐 ☹ 😜 😠 😕 😇 😎

NUTRITION

Meal 1

time eaten: _________

Meal 2

time eaten: _________

Meal 3

time eaten: _________

Meal 4

time eaten: _________

Meal 5

time eaten: _________

Hydration

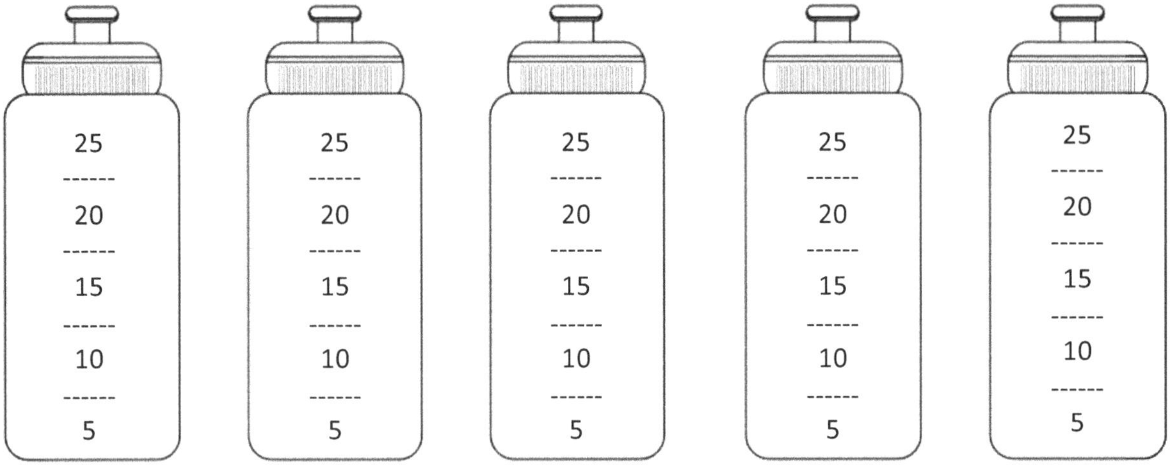

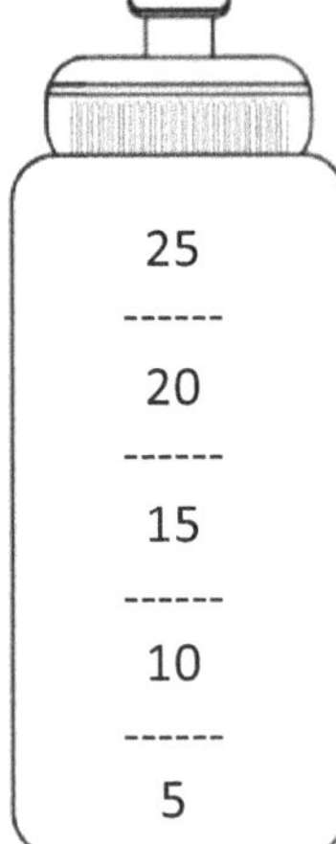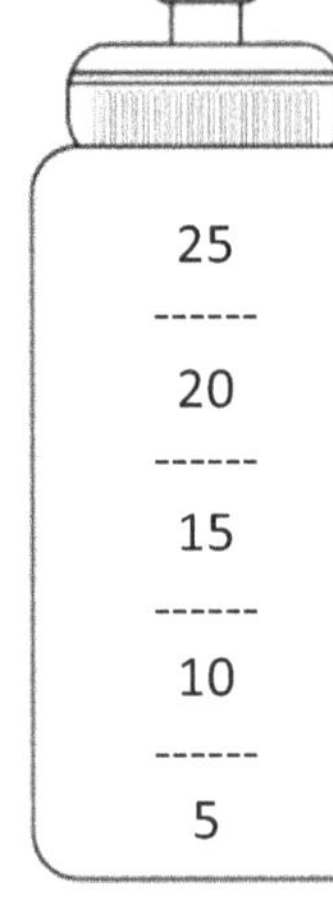

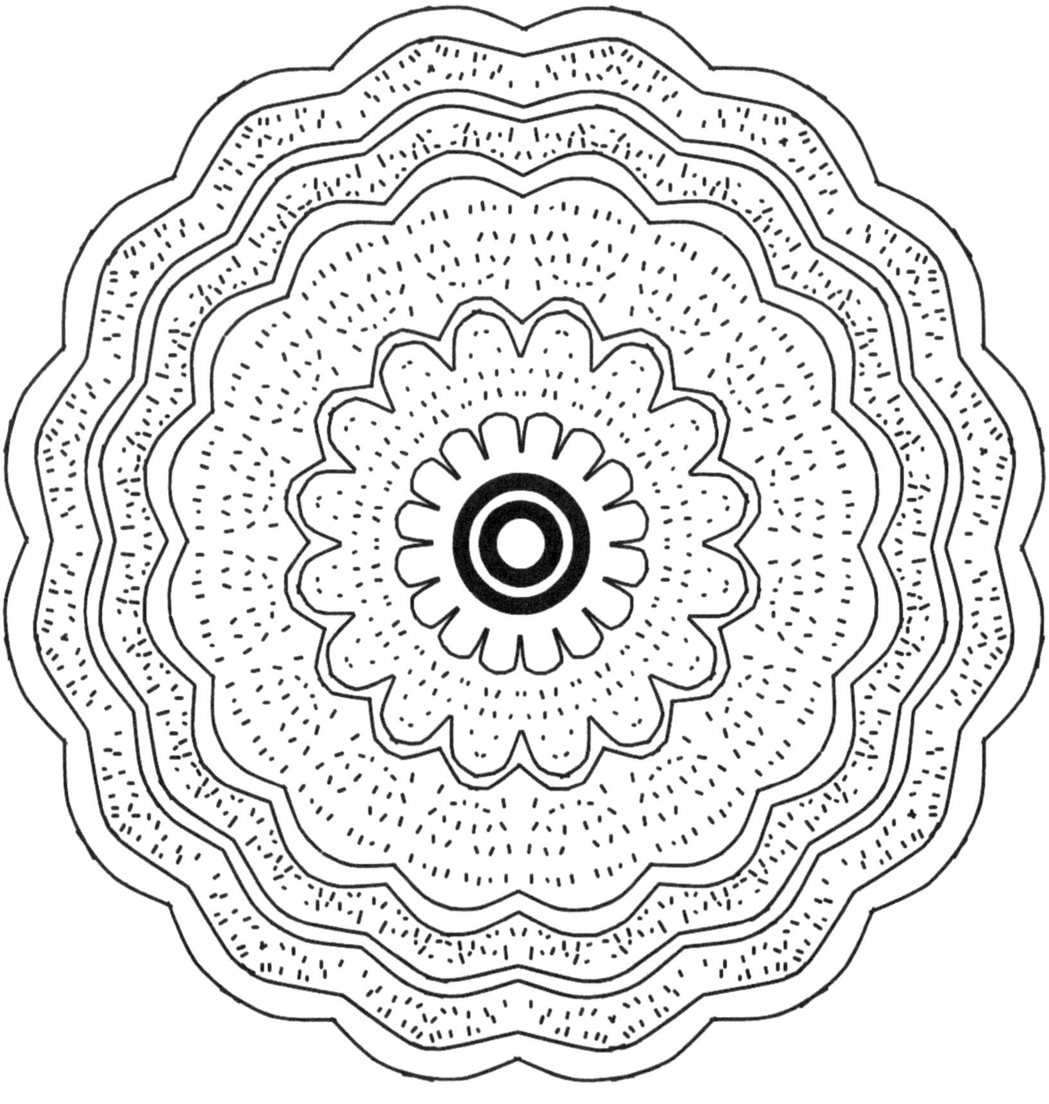

Day Eight _______

Time	
5:00	_______________________
6:00	_______________________
7:00	_______________________
8:00	_______________________
9:00	_______________________
10:00	_______________________
11:00	_______________________
Noon	_______________________
1:00	_______________________
2:00	_______________________
3:00	_______________________
4:00	_______________________
5:00	_______________________
6:00	_______________________
7:00	_______________________
8:00	_______________________
9:00	_______________________
10:00	_______________________
11:00	_______________________
Midnight	_______________________

top priorities for today 

____

____

____

____

Today's victories 🏆

What motivates you to be
the best version of you?

____

____

____

____

____

____

____

The Training

Exercise	Set 1	Set 2	Set 3	Set 4	Set 5	notes

Time started: ______________ Time ended: _______________

Location: ____

Feelings before training:

Feelings after training

NUTRITION

Meal 1
time eaten: _________

Meal 2
time eaten: _________

Meal 3
time eaten: _________

Meal 4
time eaten: _________

Meal 5
time eaten: _________

Hydration

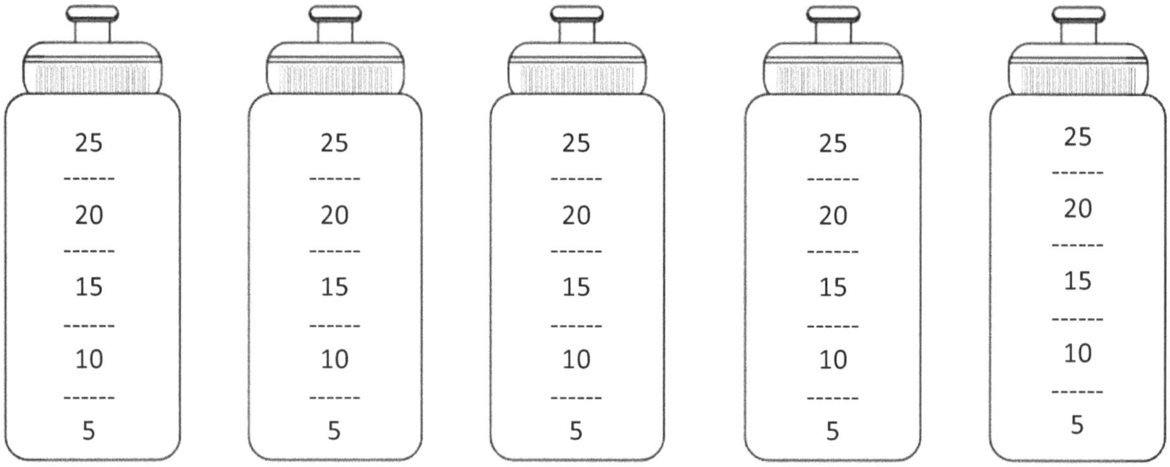

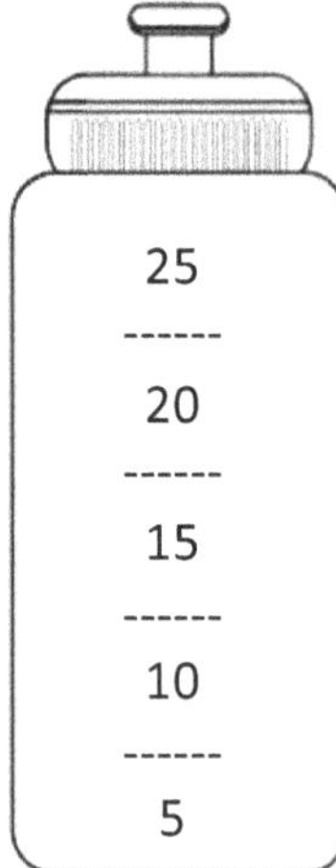 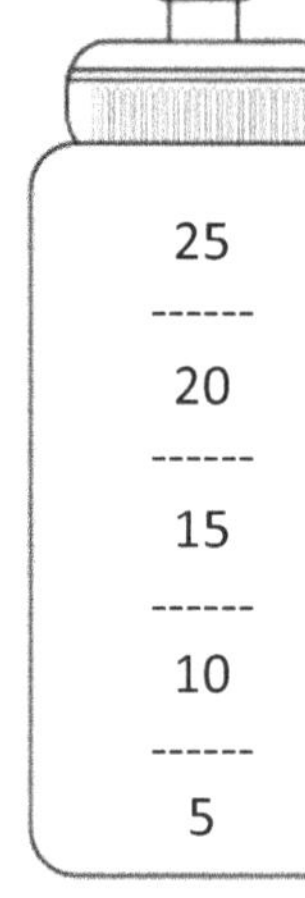

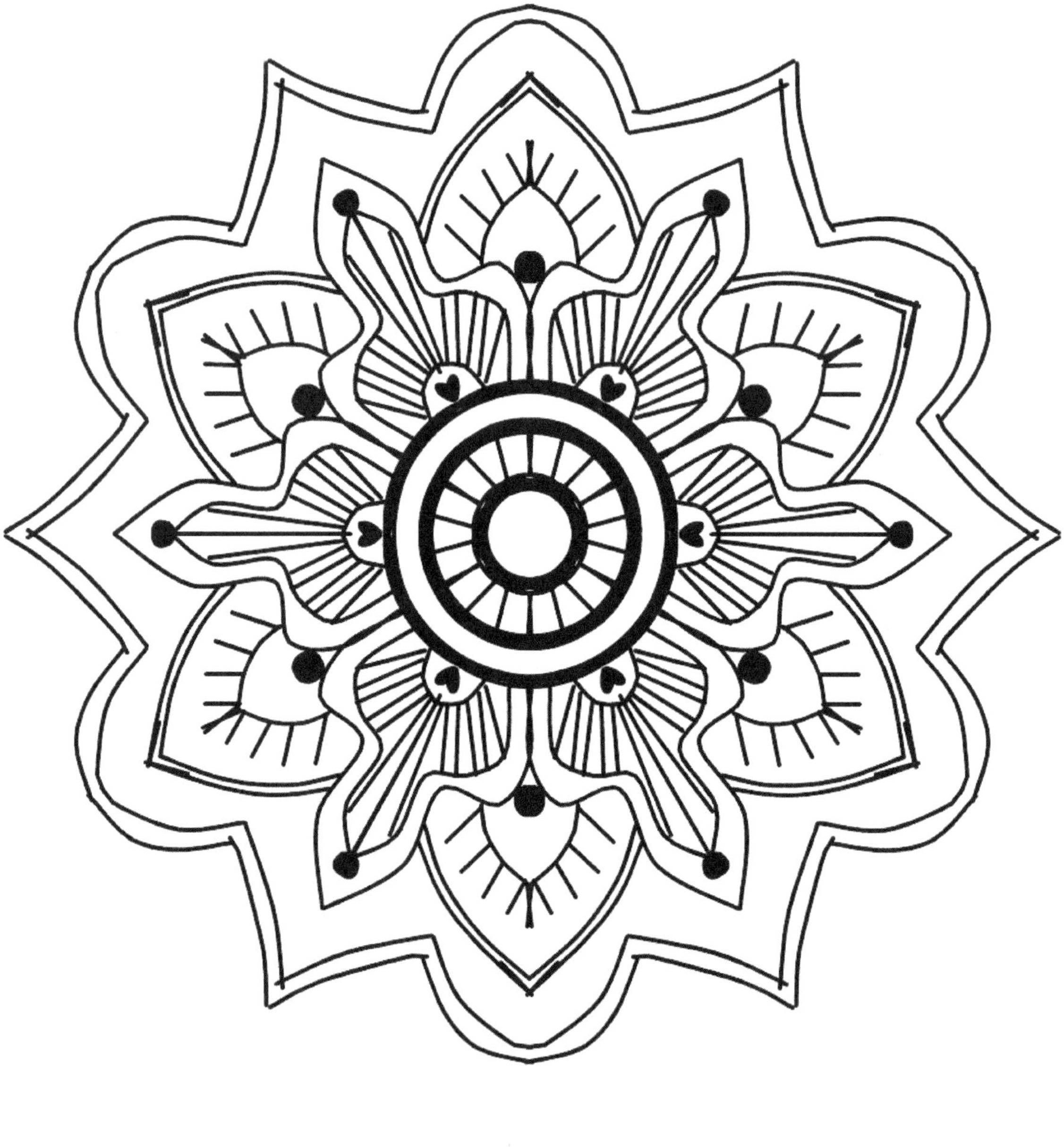

Day Nine ______

5:00 __________________	

5:00 ____________________________

6:00 ____________________________

7:00 ____________________________

8:00 ____________________________

9:00 ____________________________

10:00 __________________________

11:00 __________________________

Noon ___________________________

1:00 ____________________________

2:00 ____________________________

3:00 ____________________________

4:00 ____________________________

5:00 ____________________________

6:00 ____________________________

7:00 ____________________________

8:00 ____________________________

9:00 ____________________________

10:00 __________________________

11:00 __________________________

Midnight _____________________

top priorities for today

____

____

____

____

Today's victories

How will you be consistent this week?

____

____

____

____

____

____

The Training

Exercise	Set 1	Set 2	Set 3	Set 4	Set 5	notes

Time started: _____________ Time ended: ______________

Location: ____

Feelings before training: 😊 😐 ☹️ 😜 😠 😟 😇 😎

Feelings after training 😊 😐 ☹️ 😜 😠 😟 😇 😎

NUTRITION

Meal 1

time eaten: _________

Meal 2

time eaten: _________

Meal 3

time eaten: _________

Meal 4

time eaten: _________

Meal 5

time eaten: _________

Hydration

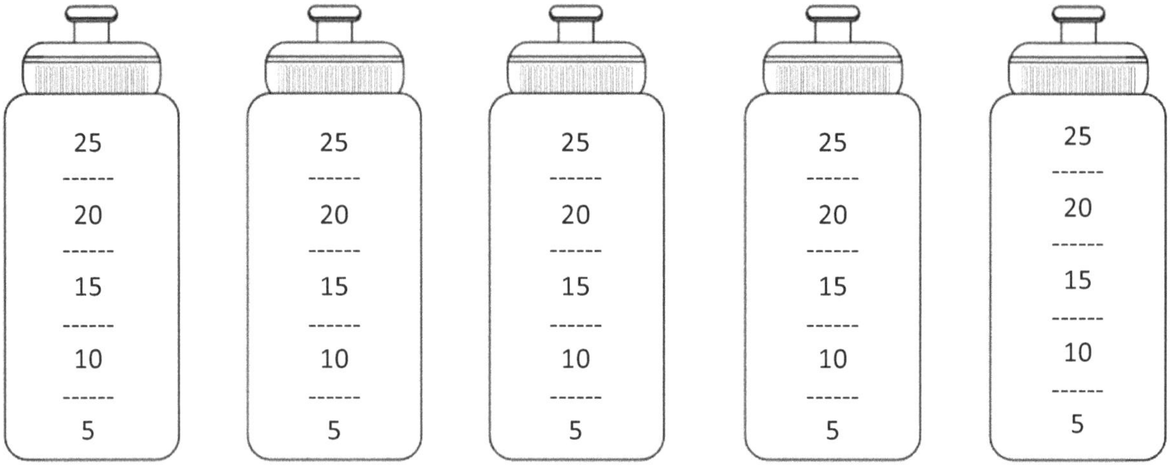

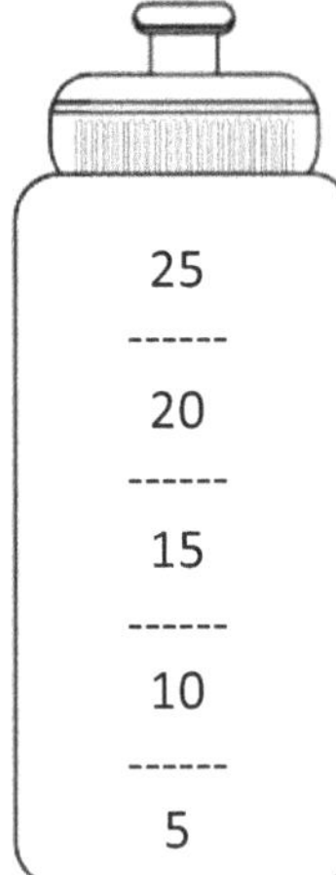 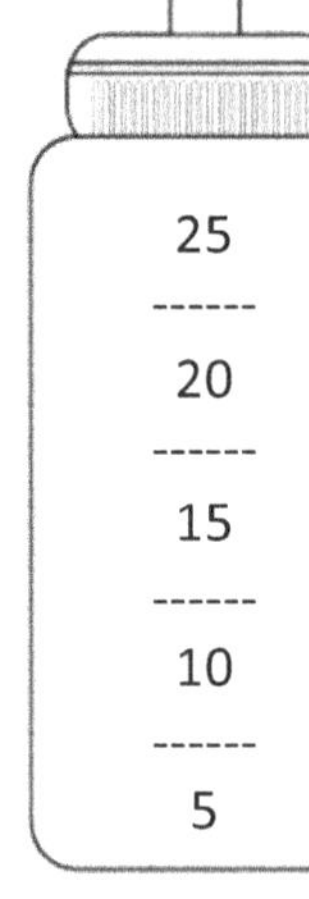

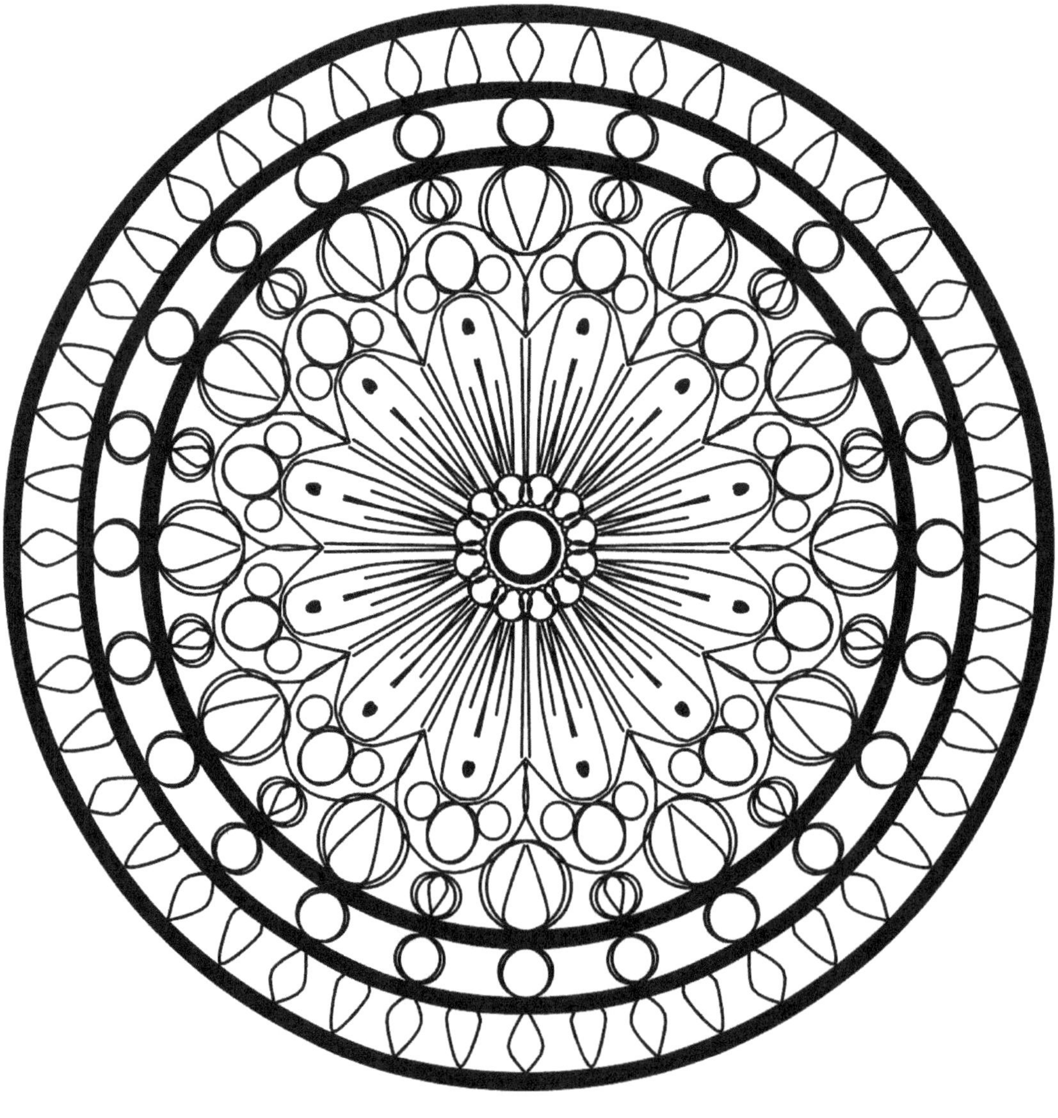

Day Ten ________

5:00 _____________________	

5:00 _____________________

6:00 _____________________

7:00 _____________________

8:00 _____________________

9:00 _____________________

10:00 _____________________

11:00 _____________________

Noon _____________________

1:00 _____________________

2:00 _____________________

3:00 _____________________

4:00 _____________________

5:00 _____________________

6:00 _____________________

7:00 _____________________

8:00 _____________________

9:00 _____________________

10:00 _____________________

11:00 _____________________

Midnight _____________________

List 5 ways you are loving.

The Training

Exercise	Set 1	Set 2	Set 3	Set 4	Set 5	notes

Time started: ________________   Time ended: ________________

Location: ____

Feelings before training:

Feelings after training

NUTRITION

Meal 1

time eaten: _________

Meal 2

time eaten: _________

Meal 3

time eaten: _________

Meal 4

time eaten: _________

Meal 5

time eaten: _________

Hydration

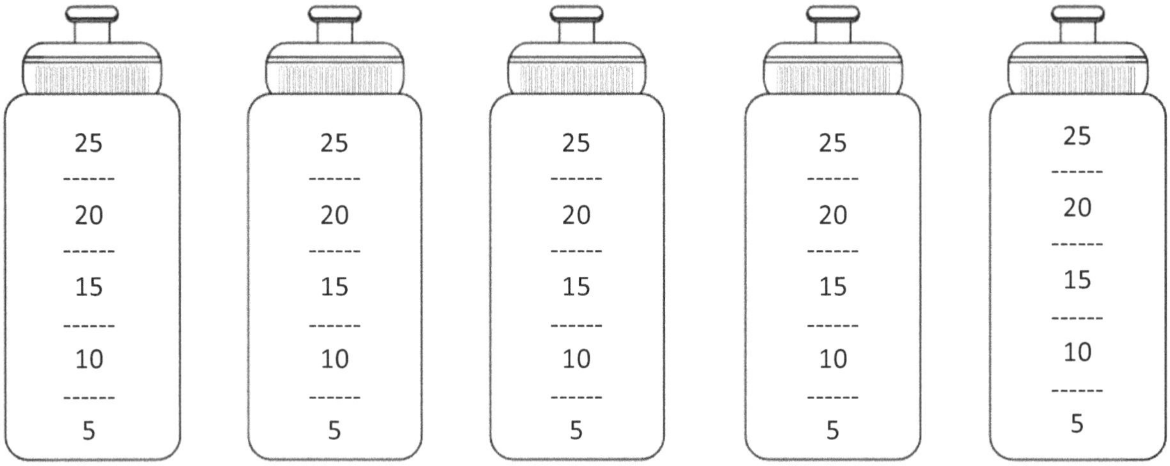

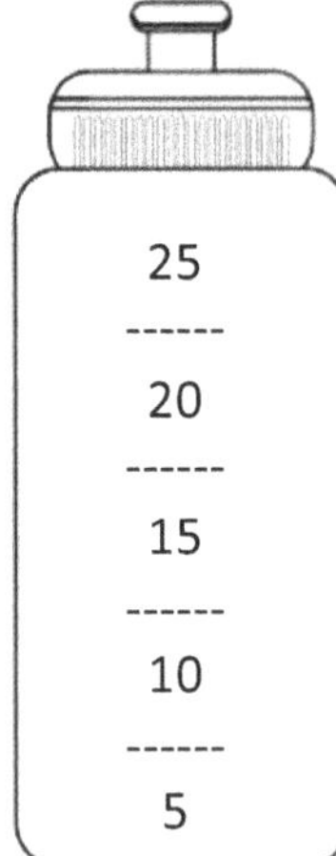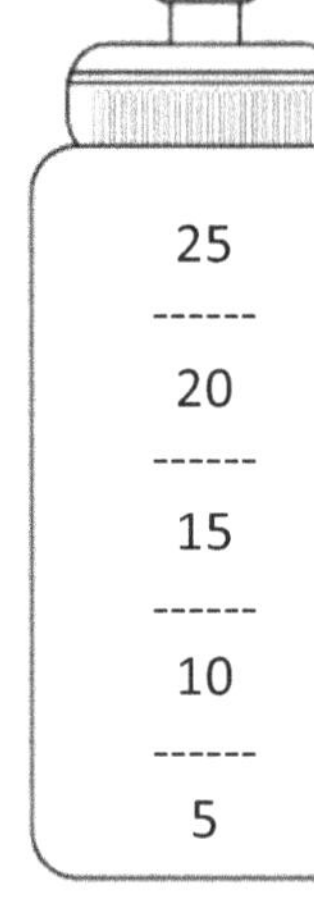

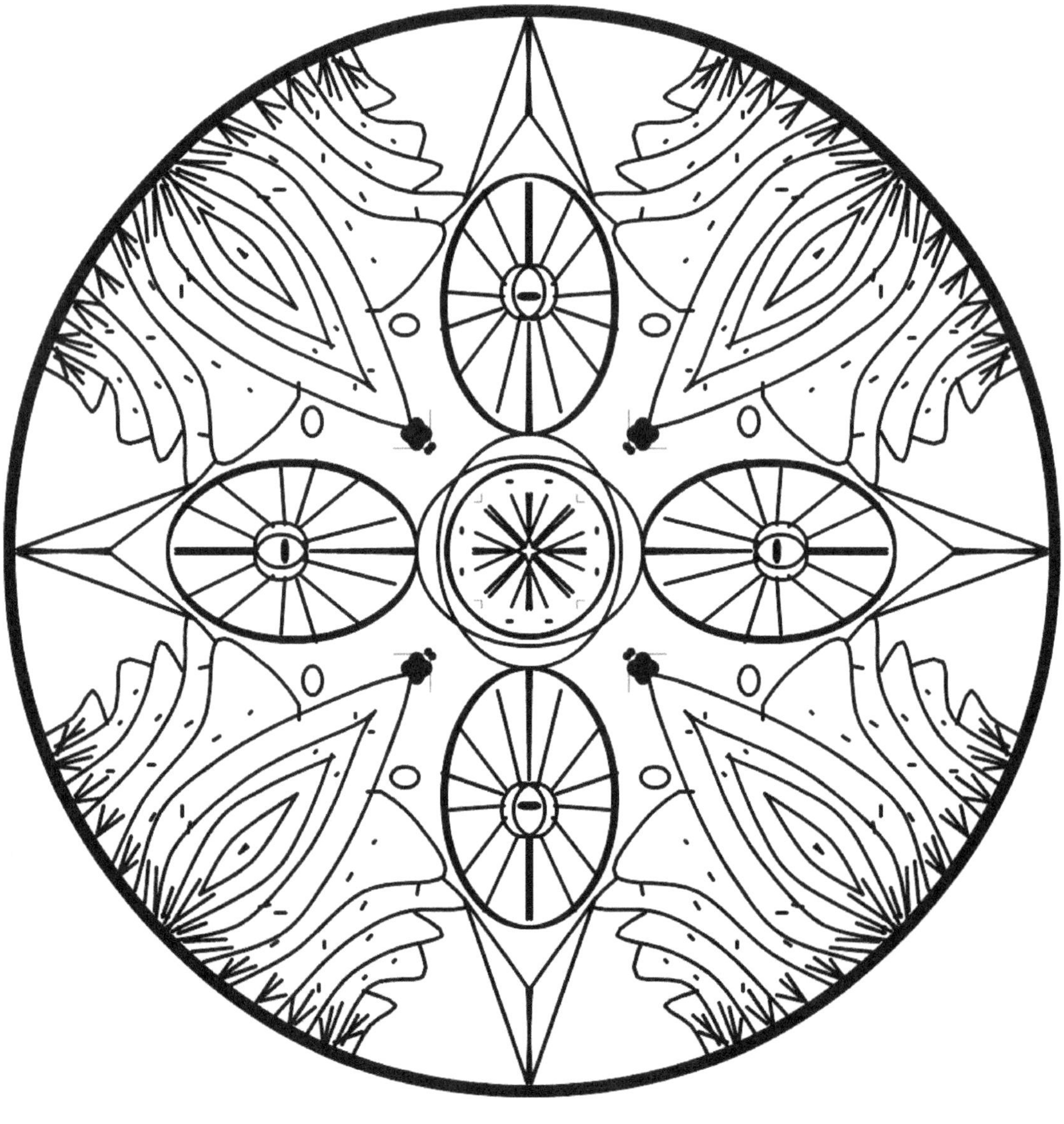

Measurements

DATE: ___________

Weight: ______

Neck ______

Shoulders _______

Chest _______

Bicep / upper arm left ________ right _______

Forearm left ________ right _______

Waist _______

Hips ______

Thighs left ________ right _____

Calf left ________ right _______

The Struggle You Are In Today, Is Developing The Strength You Need for Tomorrow.

Day Eleven ______

5:00 ______________________

6:00 ______________________

7:00 ______________________

8:00 ______________________

9:00 ______________________

10:00 ____________________

11:00 ____________________

Noon ____________________

1:00 ______________________

2:00 ______________________

3:00 ______________________

4:00 ______________________

5:00 ______________________

6:00 ______________________

7:00 ______________________

8:00 ______________________

9:00 ______________________

10:00 ____________________

11:00 ____________________

Midnight __________________

top priorities for today

Today's victories

Give out as many hugs as you can today. How many did you give?

The Training

Exercise	Set 1	Set 2	Set 3	Set 4	Set 5	notes

Time started: ______________   Time ended: ______________

Location: ____

Feelings before training: 😊 😐 🙁 😜 😣 😟 😇 😎

Feelings after training 😊 😐 🙁 😜 😣 😟 😇 😎

NUTRITION

Meal 1

time eaten: _________

Meal 2

time eaten: _________

Meal 3

time eaten: _________

Meal 4

time eaten: _________

Meal 5

time eaten: _________

Hydration

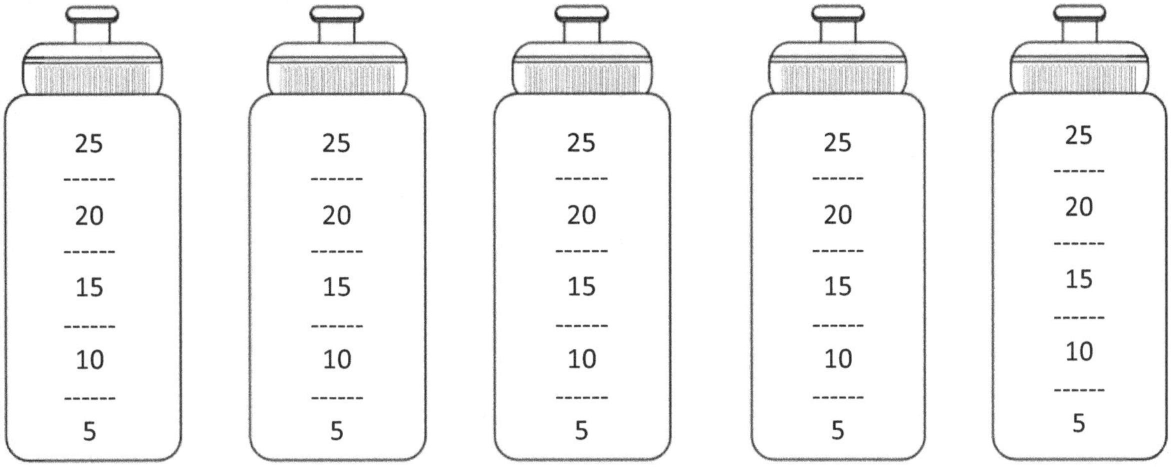

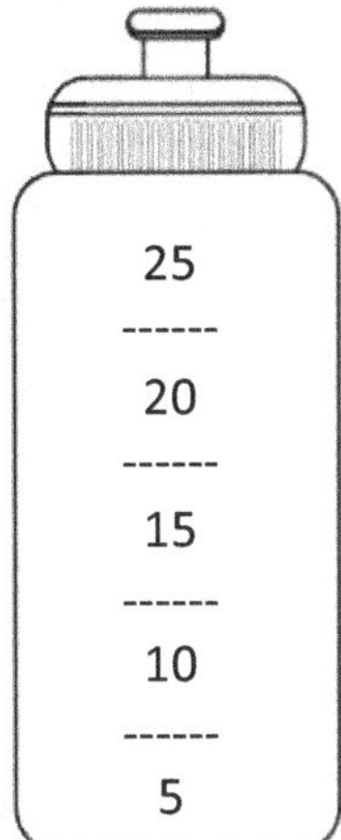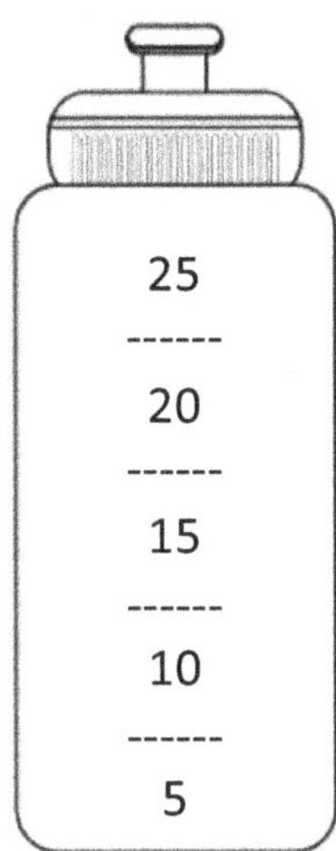

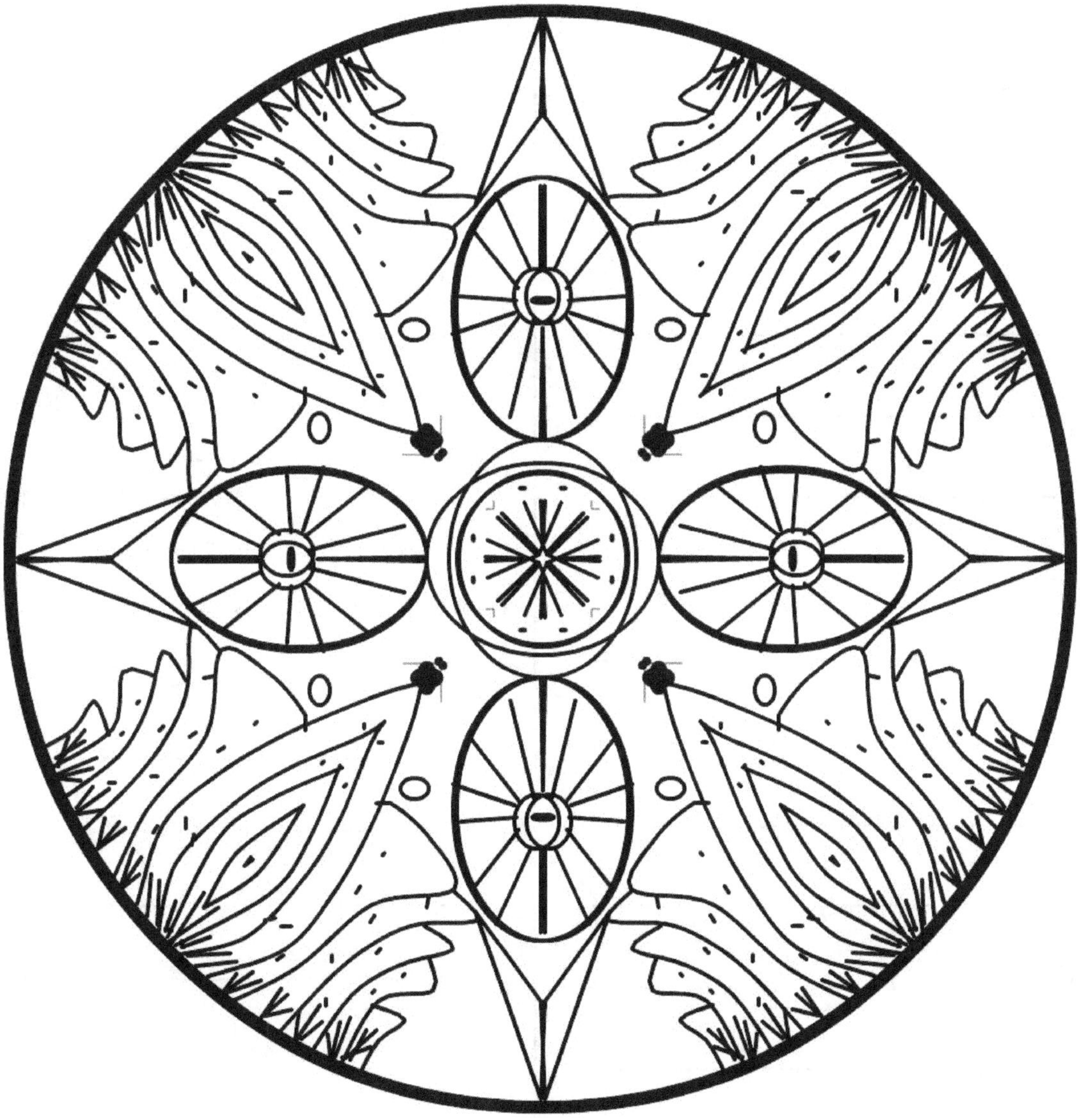

Day Twelve ______

5:00 ________________________

6:00 ________________________

7:00 ________________________

8:00 ________________________

9:00 ________________________

10:00 ________________________

11:00 ________________________

Noon ________________________

1:00 ________________________

2:00 ________________________

3:00 ________________________

4:00 ________________________

5:00 ________________________

6:00 ________________________

7:00 ________________________

8:00 ________________________

9:00 ________________________

10:00 ________________________

11:00 ________________________

Midnight ________________________

top priorities for today

Today's victories

List 4 ways you show compassion.

The Stella Society Training

Exercise	Set 1	Set 2	Set 3	Set 4	Set 5	notes

Time started: _____________   Time ended: ______________

Location: ____

Feelings before training: 😊 😐 ☹️ 😜 😠 😕 😇 😎

Feelings after training 😊 😐 ☹️ 😜 😠 😕 😇 😎

NUTRITION

Meal 1

time eaten: _________

Meal 2

time eaten: _________

Meal 3

time eaten: _________

Meal 4

time eaten: _________

Meal 5

time eaten: _________

Hydration

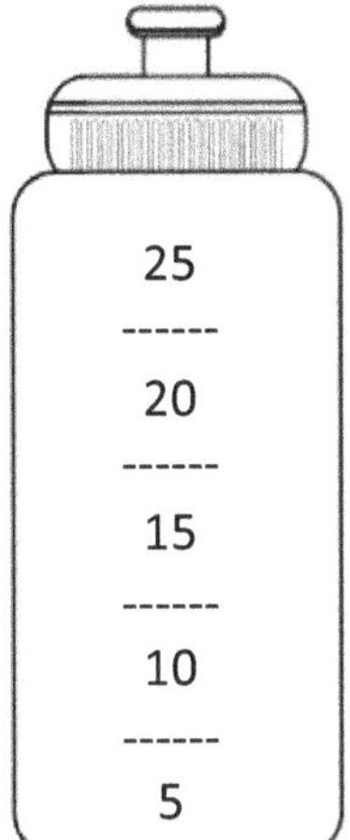
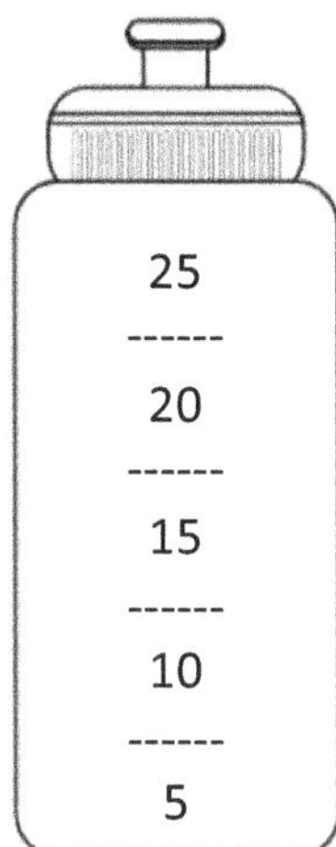
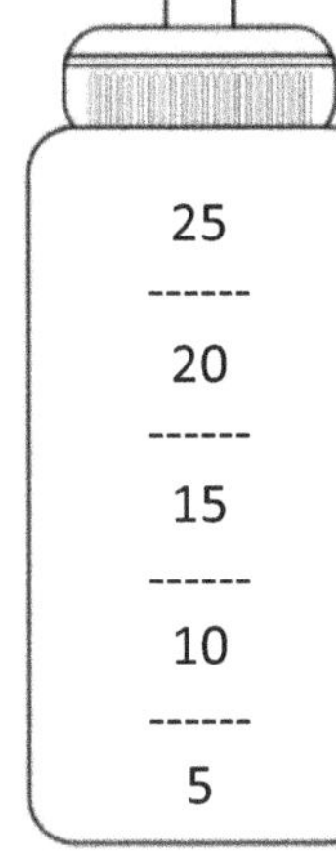
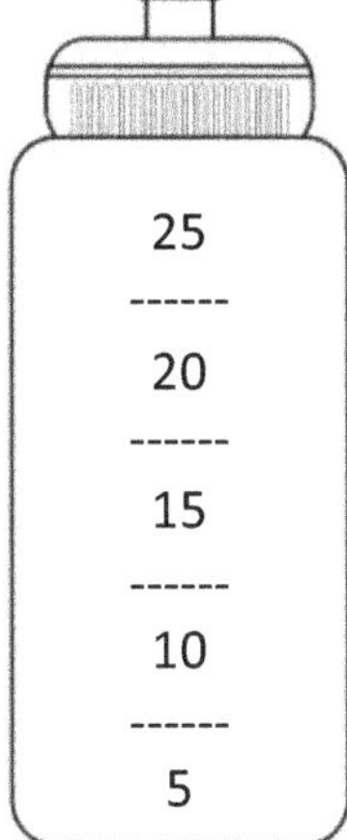
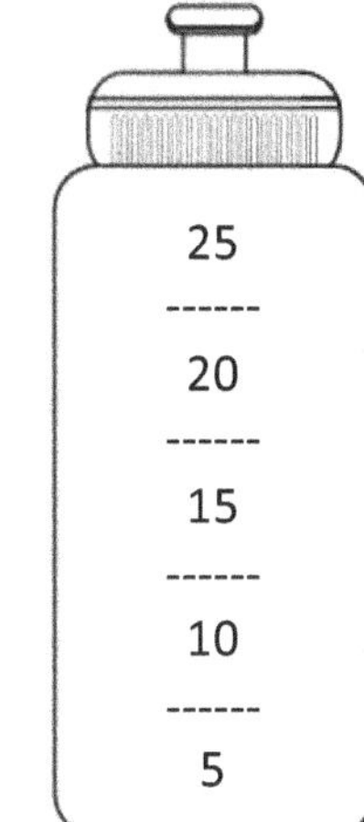

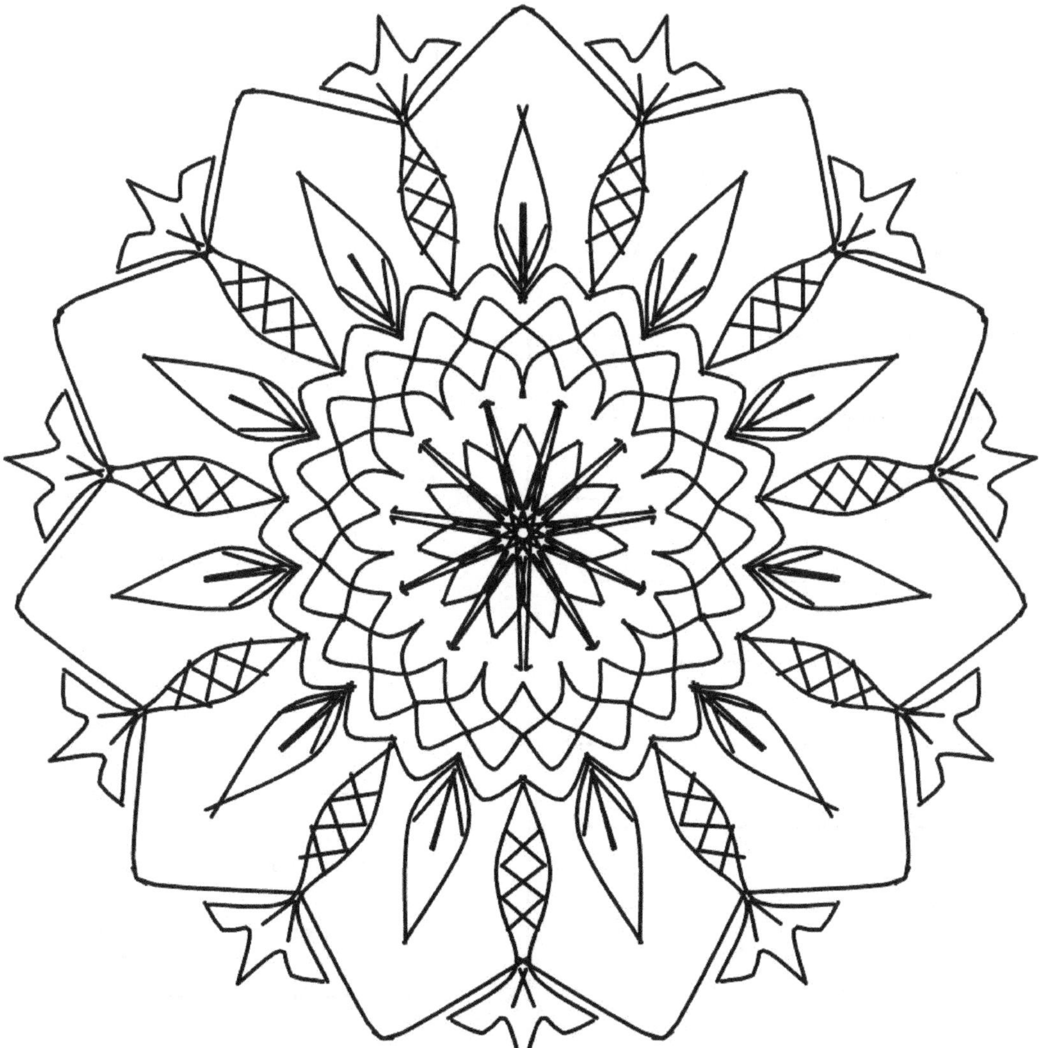

Day Thirteen __________

5:00 __________________________

6:00 __________________________

7:00 __________________________

8:00 __________________________

9:00 __________________________

10:00 _________________________

11:00 _________________________

Noon __________________________

1:00 __________________________

2:00 __________________________

3:00 __________________________

4:00 __________________________

5:00 __________________________

6:00 __________________________

7:00 __________________________

8:00 __________________________

9:00 __________________________

10:00 _________________________

11:00 _________________________

Midnight _____________________

____

____

____

____

____

Who needs roses from your garden and why?

____

____

____

____

____

____

____

The Training

Exercise	Set 1	Set 2	Set 3	Set 4	Set 5	notes

Time started: _______________   Time ended: _______________

Location: ____

Feelings before training: 🙂 😐 🙁 😜 😠 😟 😇 😎

Feelings after training 🙂 😐 🙁 😜 😠 😟 😇 😎

NUTRITION

Meal 1

time eaten: _________

Meal 2

time eaten: _________

Meal 3

time eaten: _________

Meal 4

time eaten: _________

Meal 5

time eaten: _________

Hydration

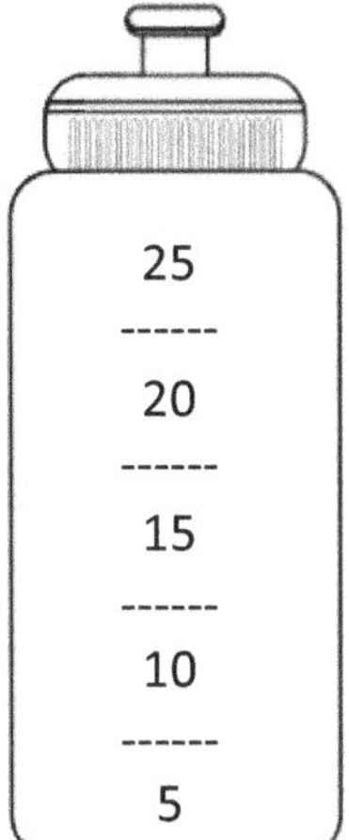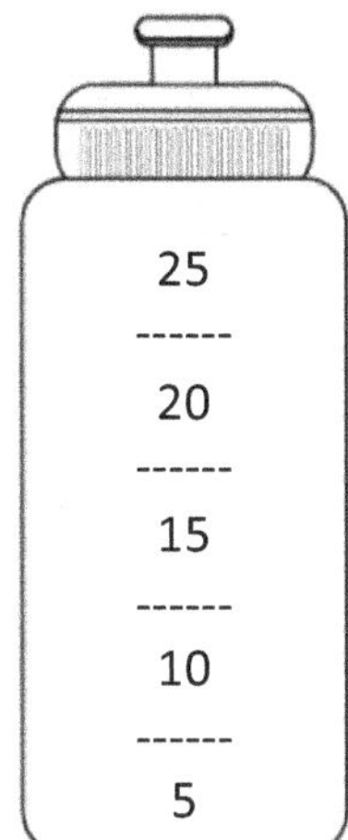

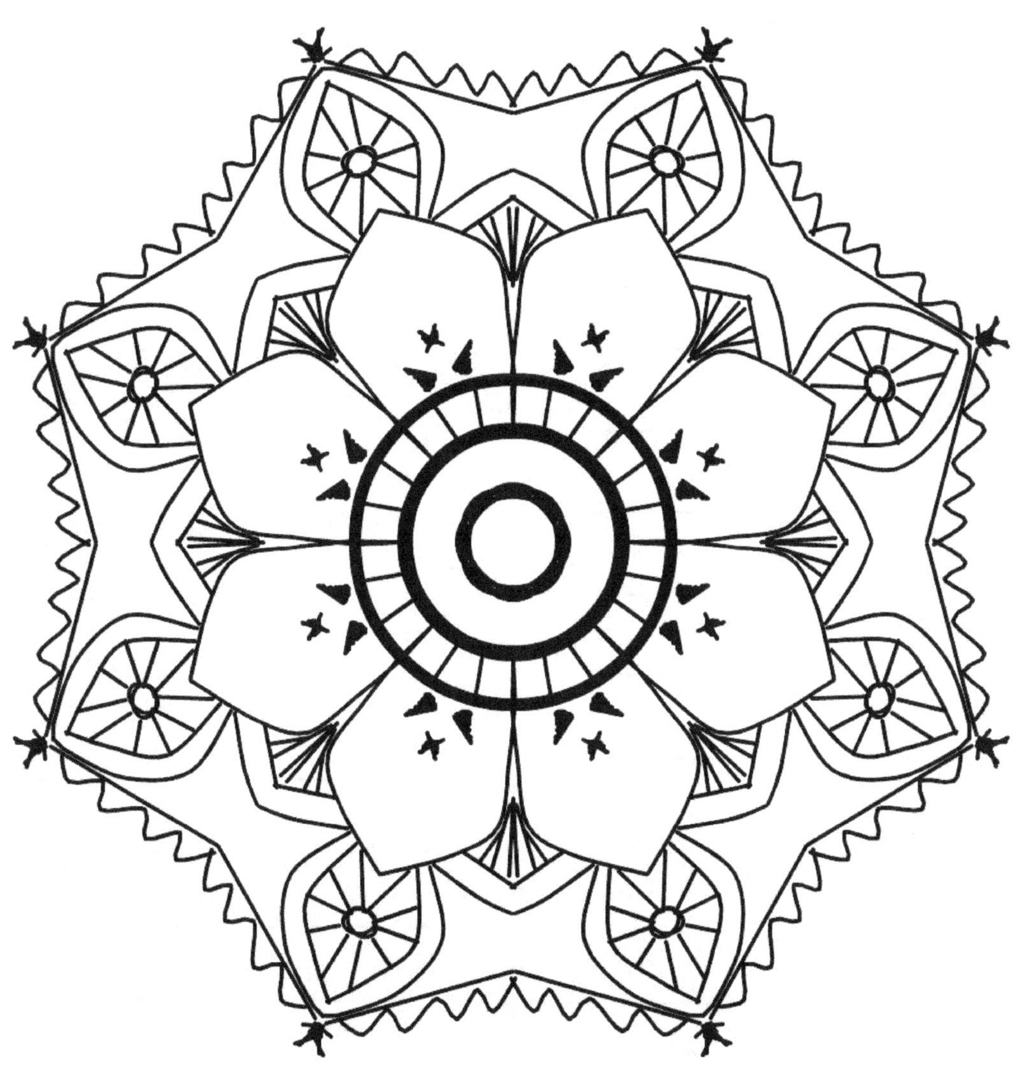

Day Fourteen ______

Schedule	
5:00	________________
6:00	________________
7:00	________________
8:00	________________
9:00	________________
10:00	________________
11:00	________________
Noon	________________
1:00	________________
2:00	________________
3:00	________________
4:00	________________
5:00	________________
6:00	________________
7:00	________________
8:00	________________
9:00	________________
10:00	________________
11:00	________________
Midnight	________________

top priorities for today

Today's victories

What should you forgive your self for?

The Training

Exercise	Set 1	Set 2	Set 3	Set 4	Set 5	notes

Time started: _____________ Time ended: _____________

Location: ____

Feelings before training:

Feelings after training

NUTRITION

Meal 1

time eaten: _________

Meal 2

time eaten: _________

Meal 3

time eaten: _________

Meal 4

time eaten: _________

Meal 5

time eaten: _________

Hydration

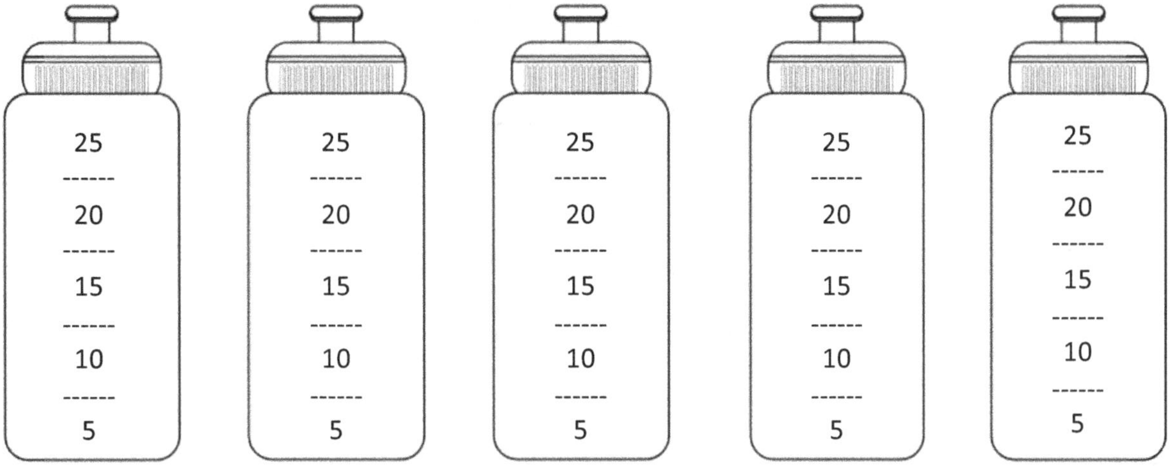

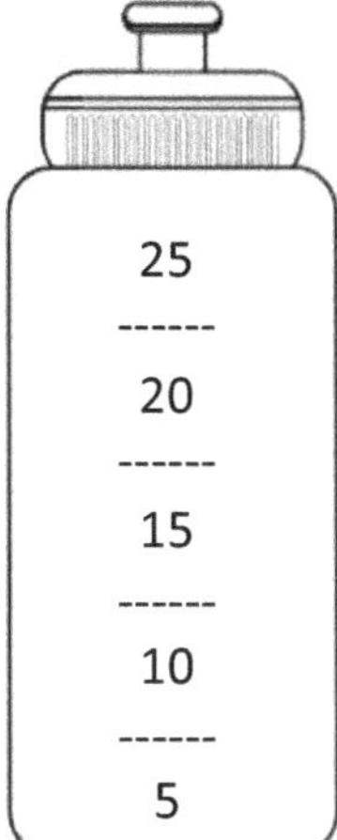
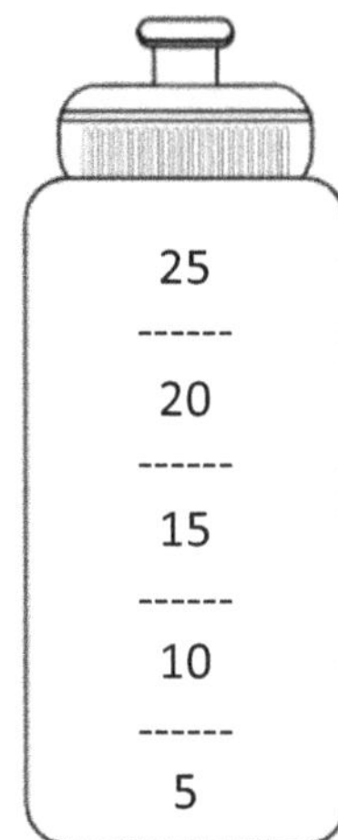

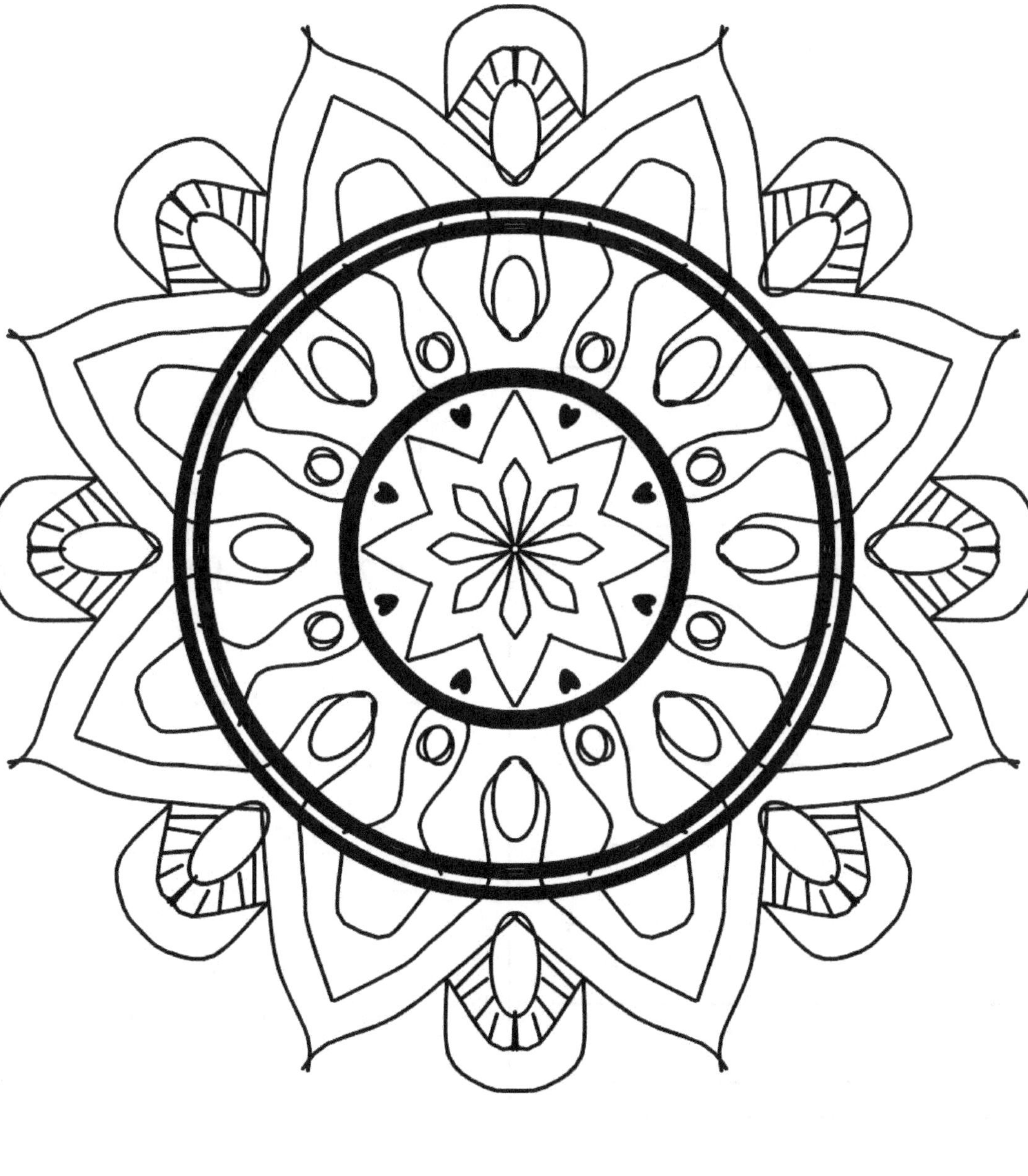

Day Fifteen _______

5:00 ______________________

6:00 ______________________

7:00 ______________________

8:00 ______________________

9:00 ______________________

10:00 ______________________

11:00 ______________________

Noon ______________________

1:00 ______________________

2:00 ______________________

3:00 ______________________

4:00 ______________________

5:00 ______________________

6:00 ______________________

7:00 ______________________

8:00 ______________________

9:00 ______________________

10:00 ______________________

11:00 ______________________

Midnight ______________________

top priorities for today

____

____

____

____

Today's victories

How will you be remarkable today?

____

____

____

____

____

The Training

Exercise	Set 1	Set 2	Set 3	Set 4	Set 5	notes

Time started: ______________ Time ended: ______________

Location: ____

Feelings before training:

Feelings after training

NUTRITION

Meal 1
time eaten: _________

Meal 2
time eaten: _________

Meal 3
time eaten: _________

Meal 4
time eaten: _________

Meal 5
time eaten: _________

Hydration

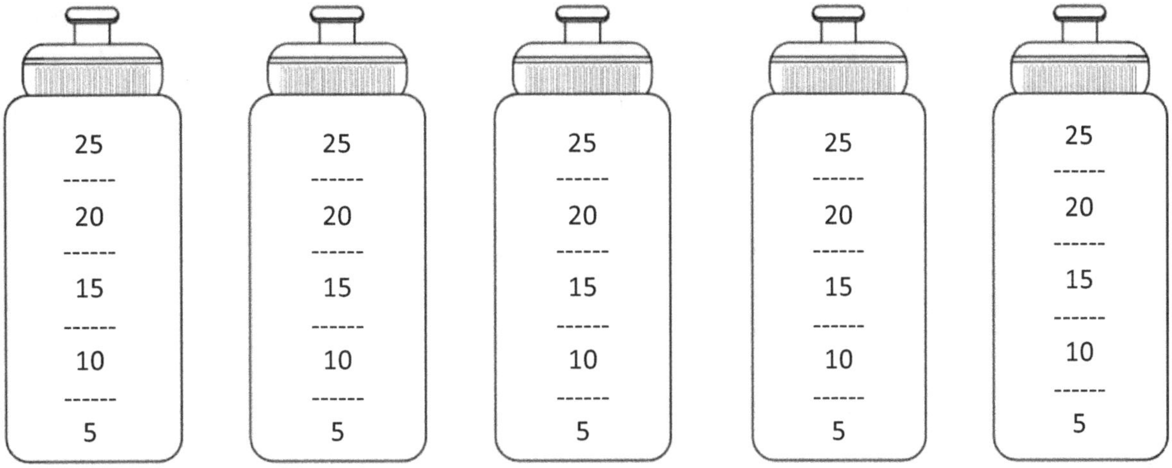

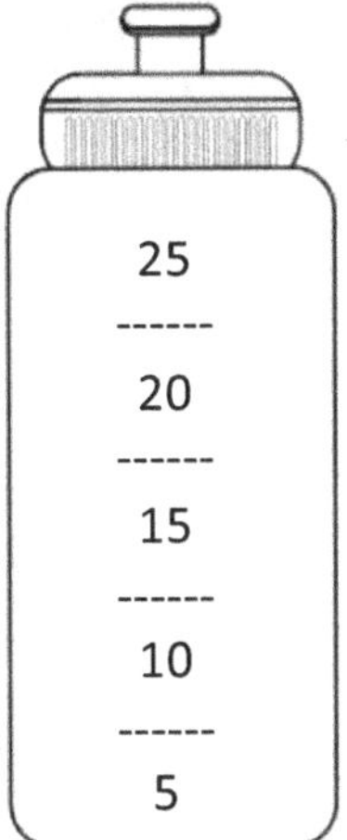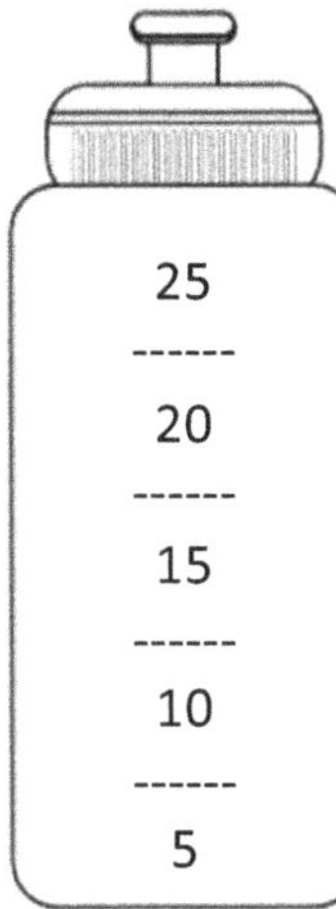

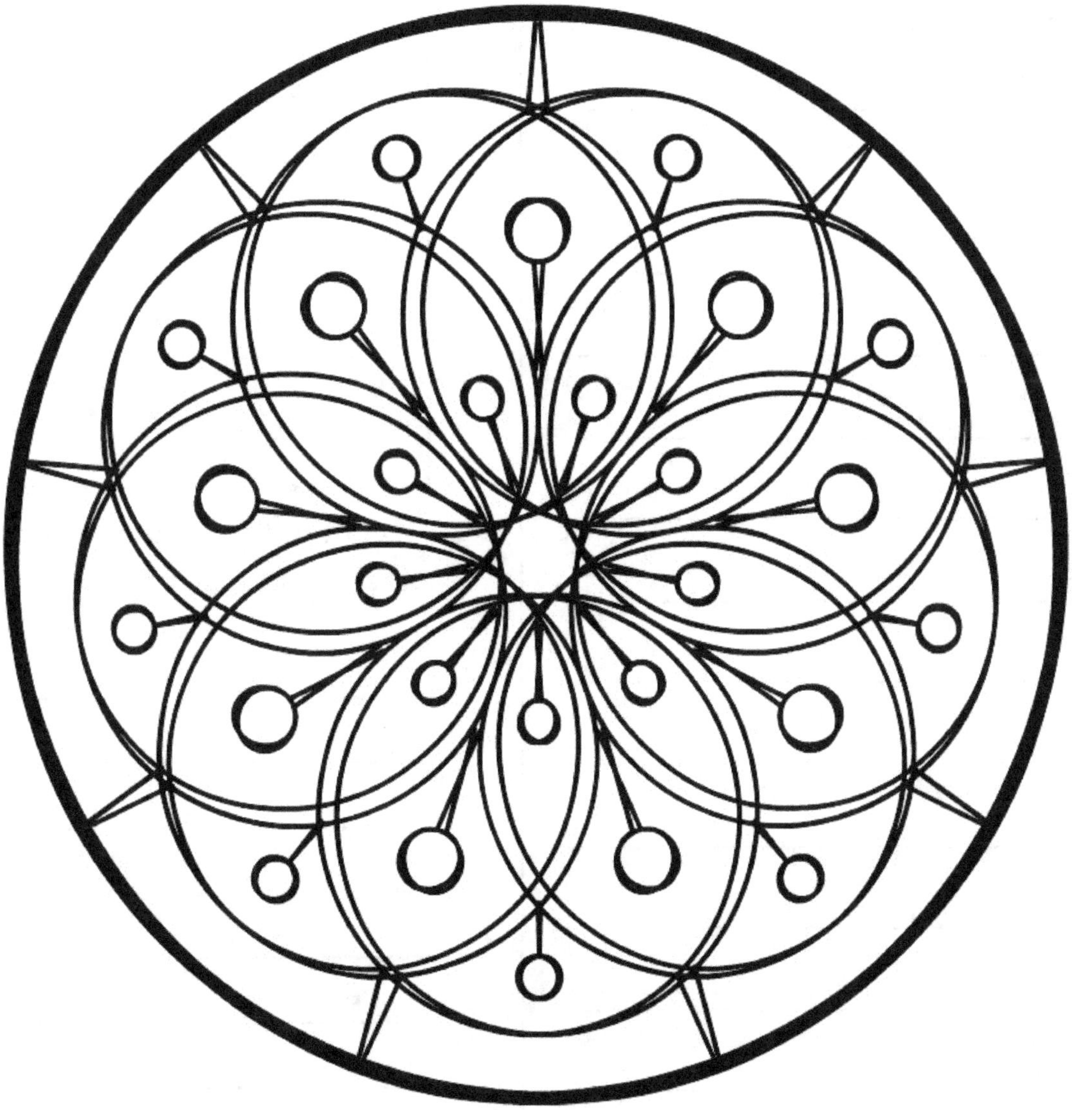

Day Sixteen _______

5:00 _______________________

6:00 _______________________

7:00 _______________________

8:00 _______________________

9:00 _______________________

10:00 ______________________

11:00 ______________________

Noon _______________________

1:00 _______________________

2:00 _______________________

3:00 _______________________

4:00 _______________________

5:00 _______________________

6:00 _______________________

7:00 _______________________

8:00 _______________________

9:00 _______________________

10:00 ______________________

11:00 ______________________

Midnight ____________________

top priorities for today

____

____

____

____

Today's victories

Watch the sunset and list 5 places you want to see it happen?

____

____

____

____

____

____

The Stella Society Training

Exercise	Set 1	Set 2	Set 3	Set 4	Set 5	notes

Time started: _____________   Time ended: _____________

Location: ____

Feelings before training: 😊 😐 ☹️ 😜 😠 😟 😇 😎

Feelings after training 😊 😐 ☹️ 😜 😠 😟 😇 😎

NUTRITION

Meal 1
time eaten: _________

Meal 2
time eaten: _________

Meal 3
time eaten: _________

Meal 4
time eaten: _________

Meal 5
time eaten: _________

Hydration

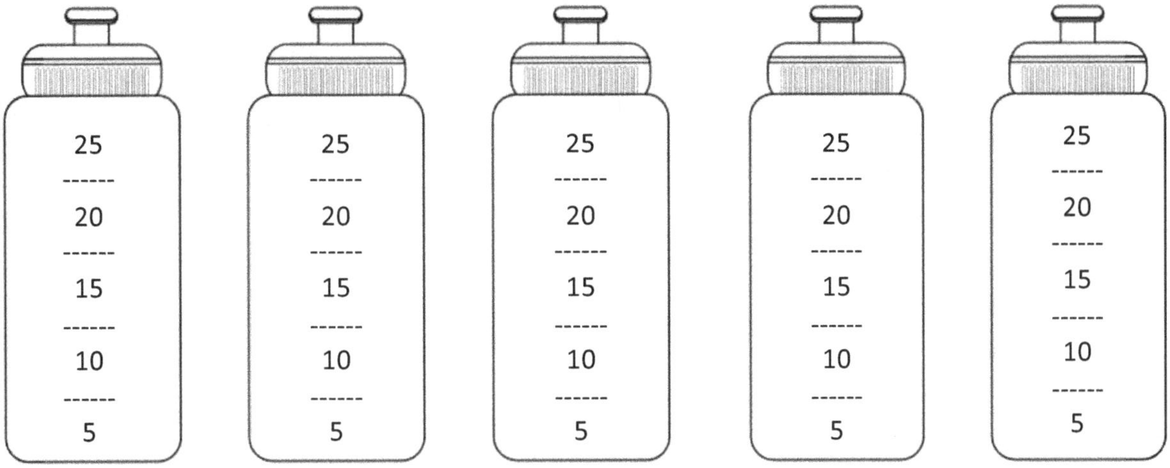

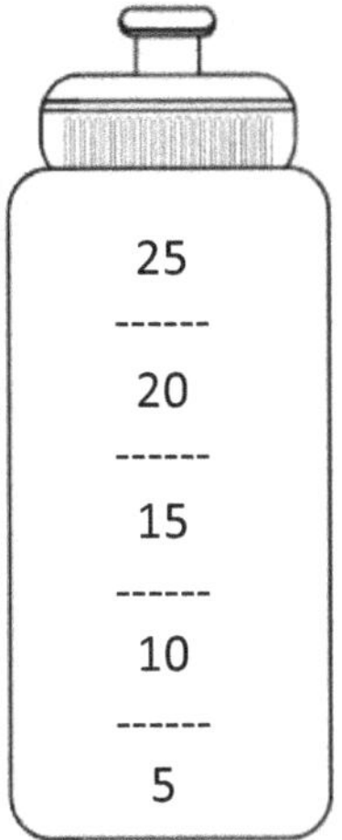
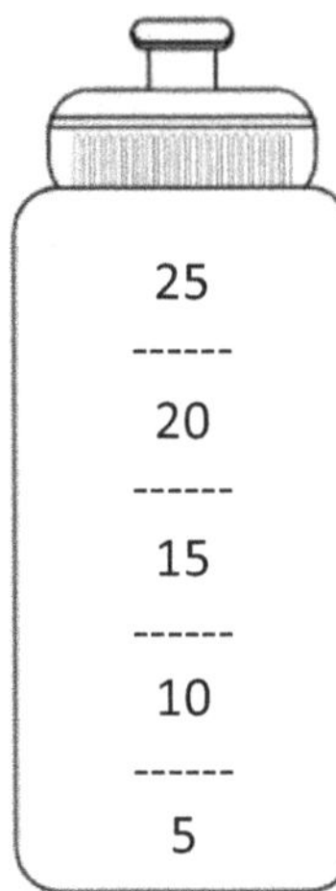
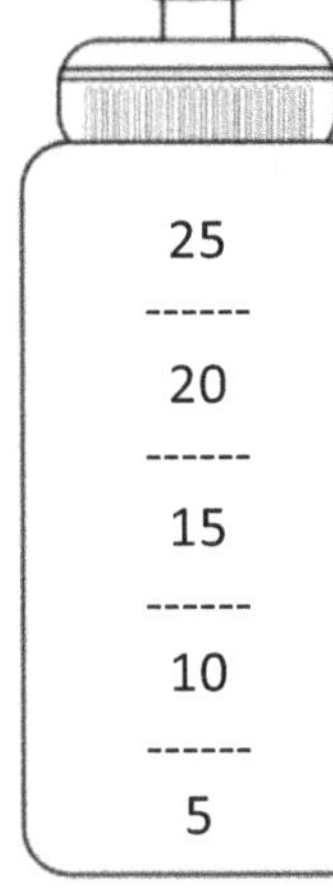
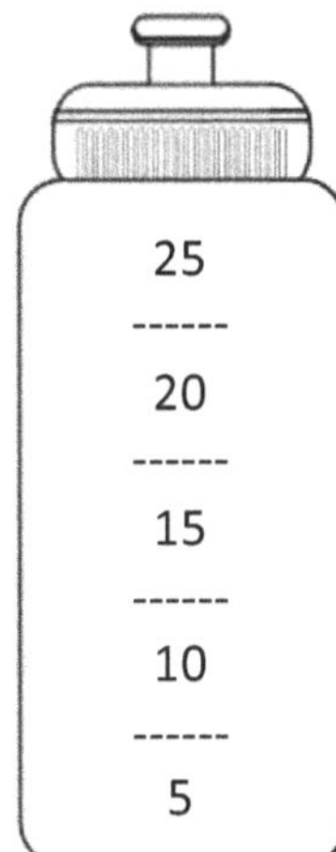

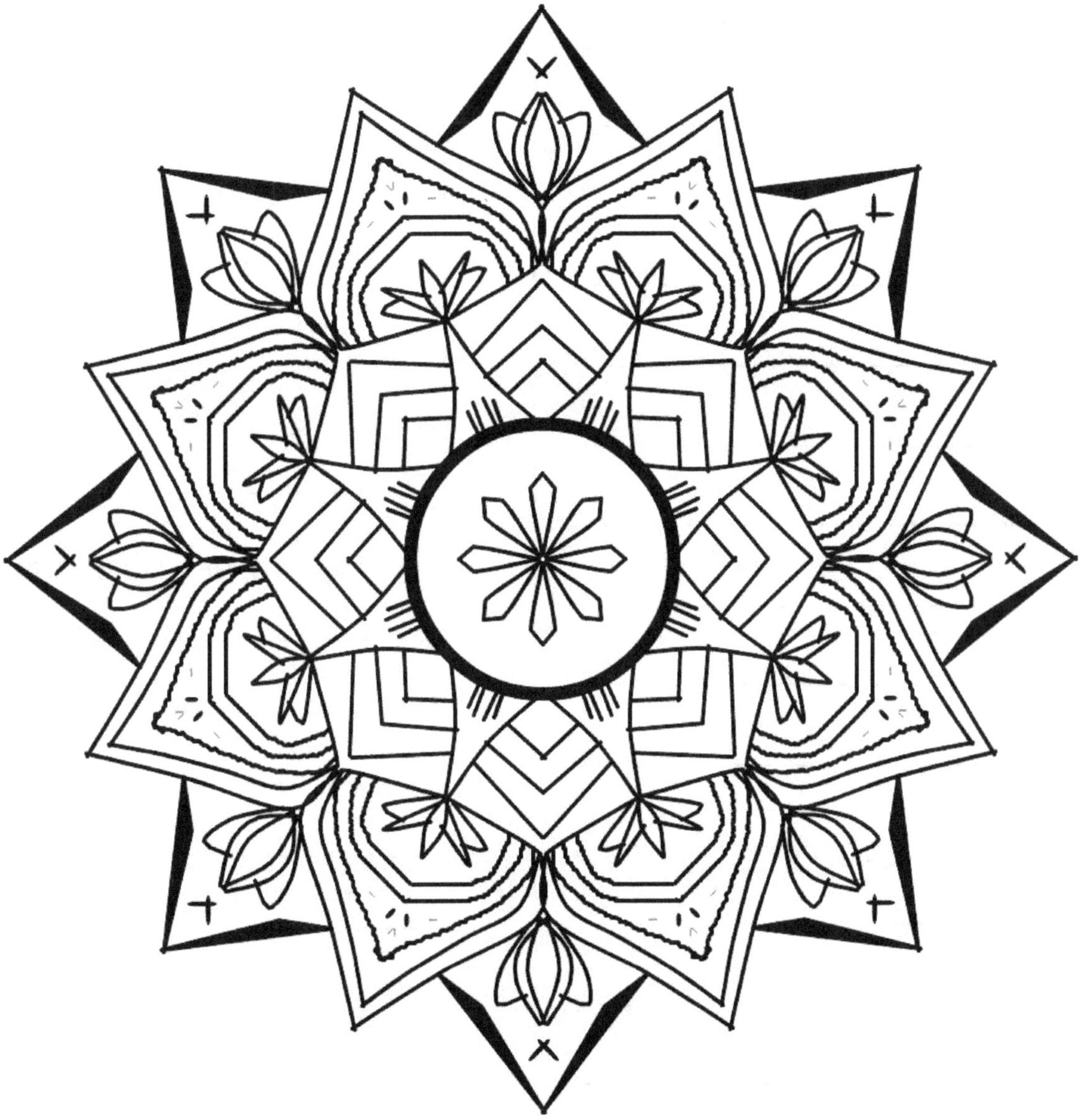

Day Seventeen ________

Time	
5:00	___________________
6:00	___________________
7:00	___________________
8:00	___________________
9:00	___________________
10:00	___________________
11:00	___________________
Noon	___________________
1:00	___________________
2:00	___________________
3:00	___________________
4:00	___________________
5:00	___________________
6:00	___________________
7:00	___________________
8:00	___________________
9:00	___________________
10:00	___________________
11:00	___________________
Midnight	___________________

top priorities for today

____

____

____

____

Today's victories

What makes you happy?

____

____

____

____

____

____

The Training

<table>
<tr><th>Exercise</th><th>Set 1</th><th>Set 2</th><th>Set 3</th><th>Set 4</th><th>Set 5</th><th>notes</th></tr>
<tr><td></td><td></td><td></td><td></td><td></td><td></td><td></td></tr>
<tr><td></td><td></td><td></td><td></td><td></td><td></td><td></td></tr>
<tr><td></td><td></td><td></td><td></td><td></td><td></td><td></td></tr>
<tr><td></td><td></td><td></td><td></td><td></td><td></td><td></td></tr>
<tr><td></td><td></td><td></td><td></td><td></td><td></td><td></td></tr>
<tr><td></td><td></td><td></td><td></td><td></td><td></td><td></td></tr>
</table>

Time started: _____________   Time ended: _____________

Location: ____

Feelings before training:

Feelings after training

NUTRITION

Meal 1

time eaten: _________

Meal 2

time eaten: _________

Meal 3

time eaten: _________

Meal 4

time eaten: _________

Meal 5

time eaten: _________

Hydration

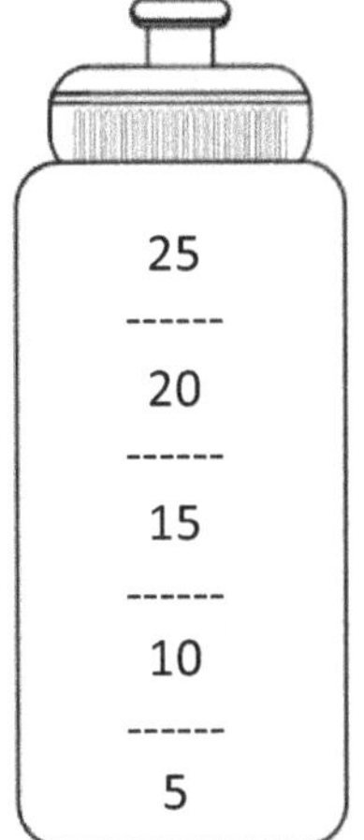
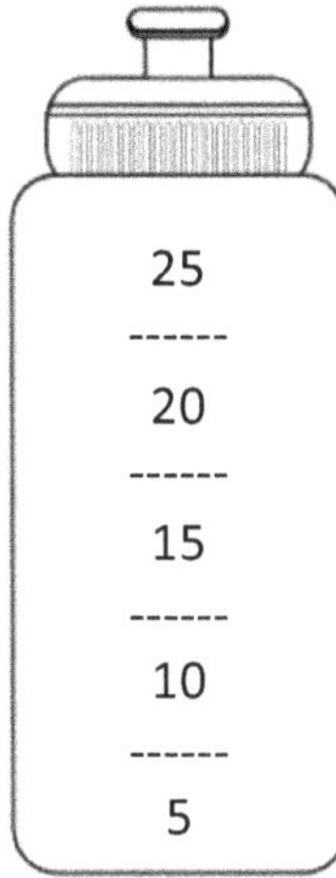
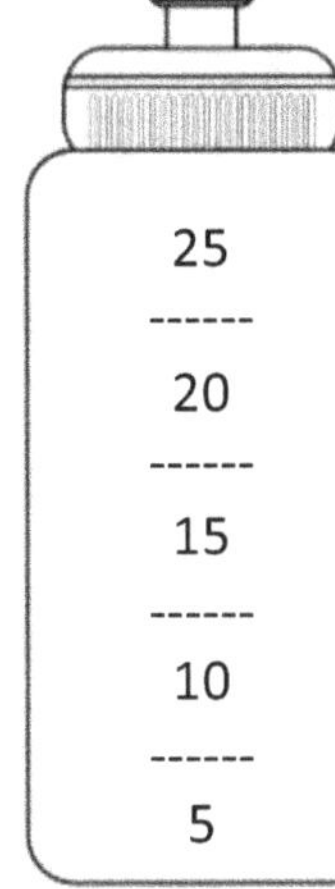
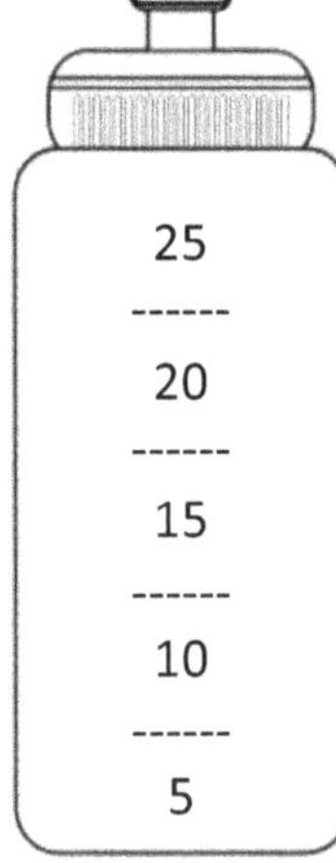
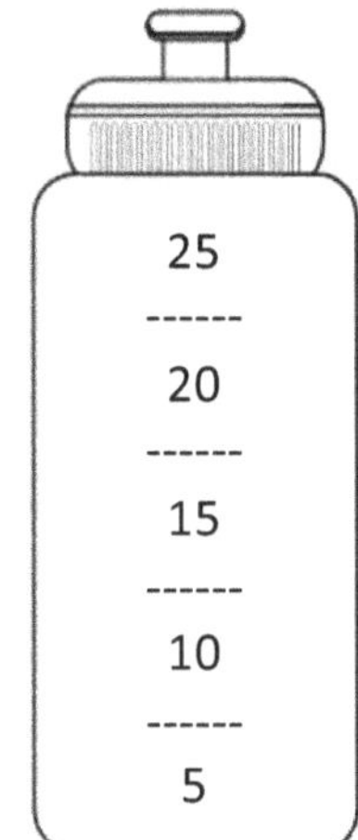

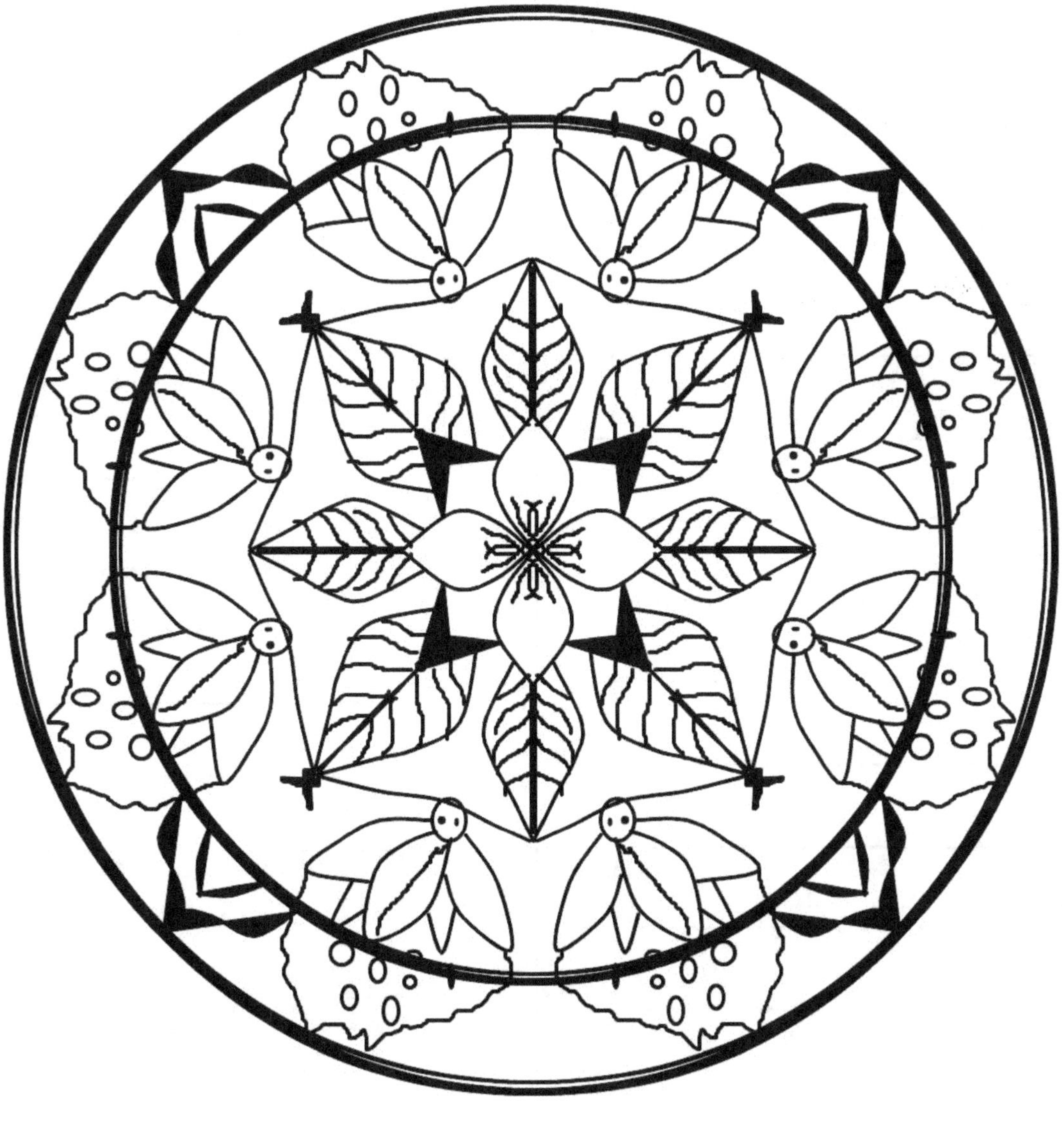

Day Eighteen ________

5:00 ________________________

6:00 ________________________

7:00 ________________________

8:00 ________________________

9:00 ________________________

10:00 ______________________

11:00 ______________________

Noon ______________________

1:00 ________________________

2:00 ________________________

3:00 ________________________

4:00 ________________________

5:00 ________________________

6:00 ________________________

7:00 ________________________

8:00 ________________________

9:00 ________________________

10:00 ______________________

11:00 ______________________

Midnight __________________

Today's victories

Where will you shine your light this week?

The Stella Society Training

Exercise	Set 1	Set 2	Set 3	Set 4	Set 5	notes

Time started: _______________ Time ended: _______________

Location: ____

Feelings before training:

Feelings after training

NUTRITION

Meal 1

time eaten: _________

Meal 2

time eaten: _________

Meal 3

time eaten: _________

Meal 4

time eaten: _________

Meal 5

time eaten: _________

Hydration

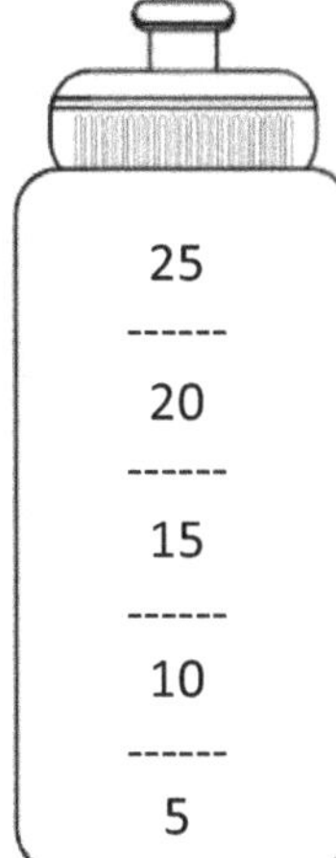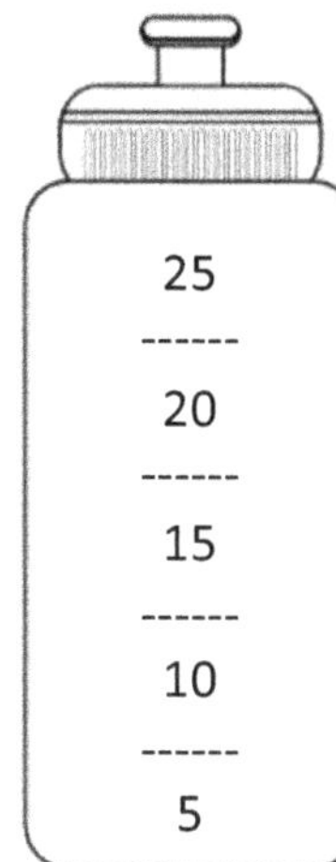

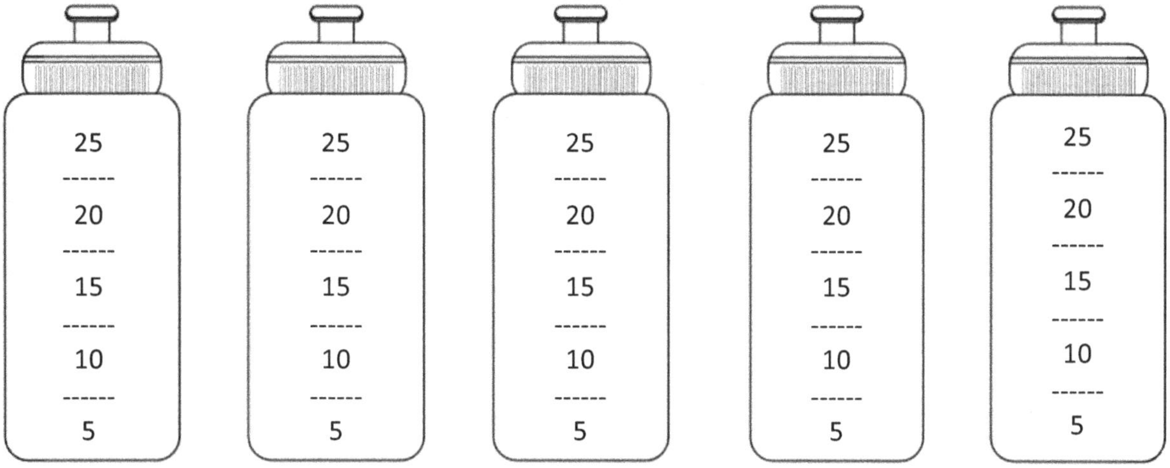

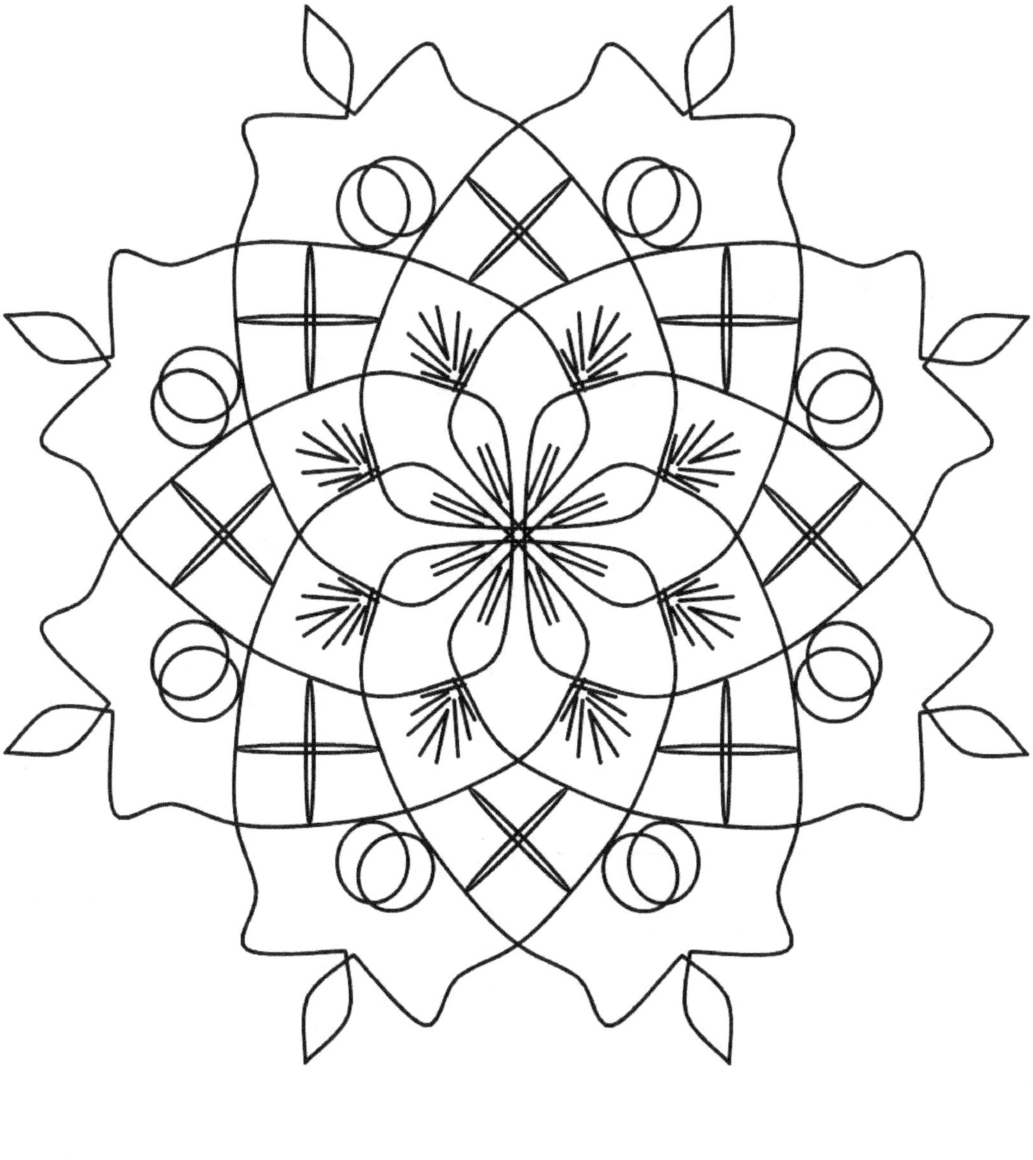

25	25	25	25	25
20	20	20	20	20
15	15	15	15	15
10	10	10	10	10
5	5	5	5	5

Day Nineteen _______

5:00 _______________________

6:00 _______________________

7:00 _______________________

8:00 _______________________

9:00 _______________________

10:00 ______________________

11:00 ______________________

Noon _______________________

1:00 _______________________

2:00 _______________________

3:00 _______________________

4:00 _______________________

5:00 _______________________

6:00 _______________________

7:00 _______________________

8:00 _______________________

9:00 _______________________

10:00 ______________________

11:00 ______________________

Midnight ___________________

____

____

____

____

You are charming, how will
you show it?

____

____

____

____

____

____

The Training

Exercise	Set 1	Set 2	Set 3	Set 4	Set 5	notes

Time started: ______________   Time ended: ______________

Location: ____

Feelings before training:

Feelings after training

NUTRITION

Meal 1

time eaten: _________

Meal 2

time eaten: _________

Meal 3

time eaten: _________

Meal 4

time eaten: _________

Meal 5

time eaten: _________

Hydration

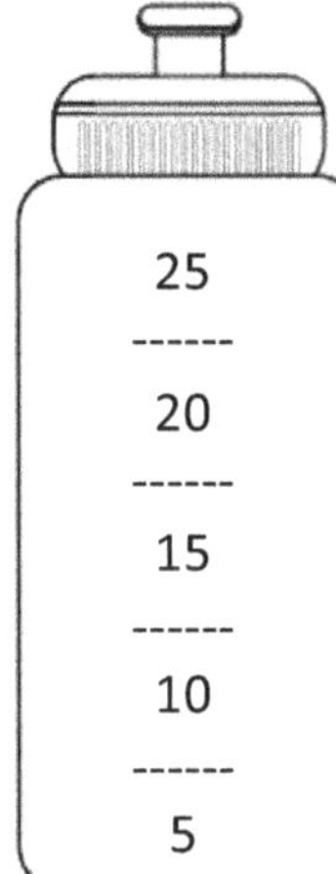

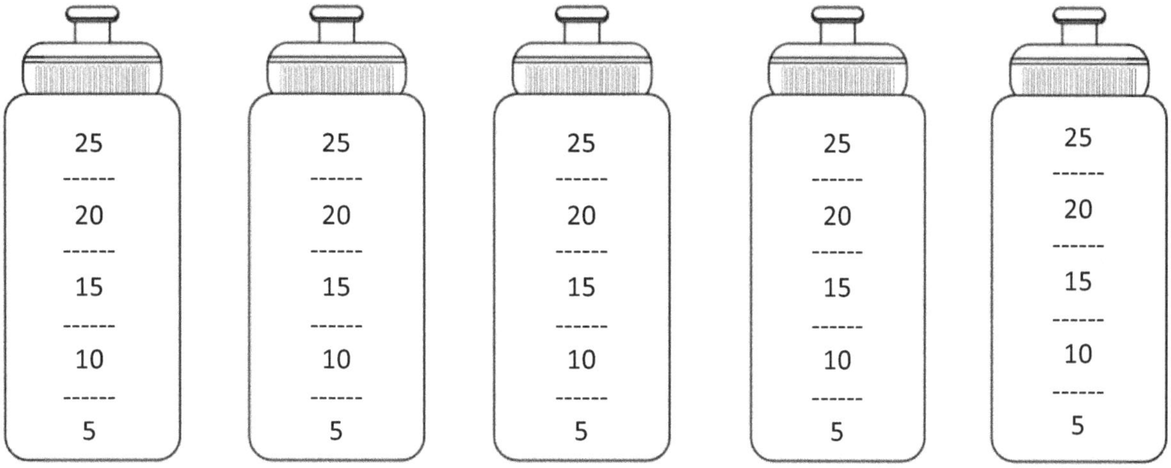

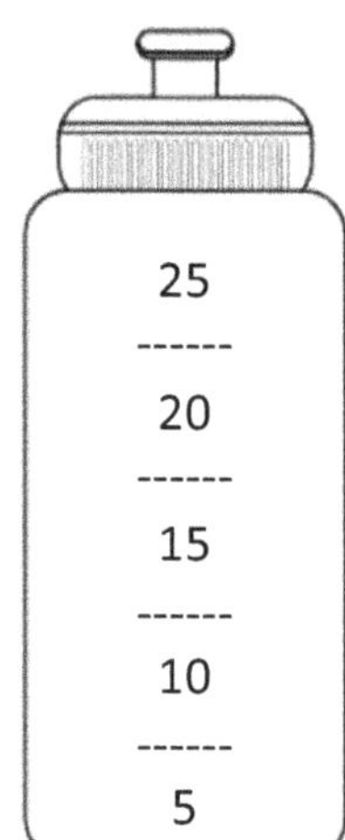

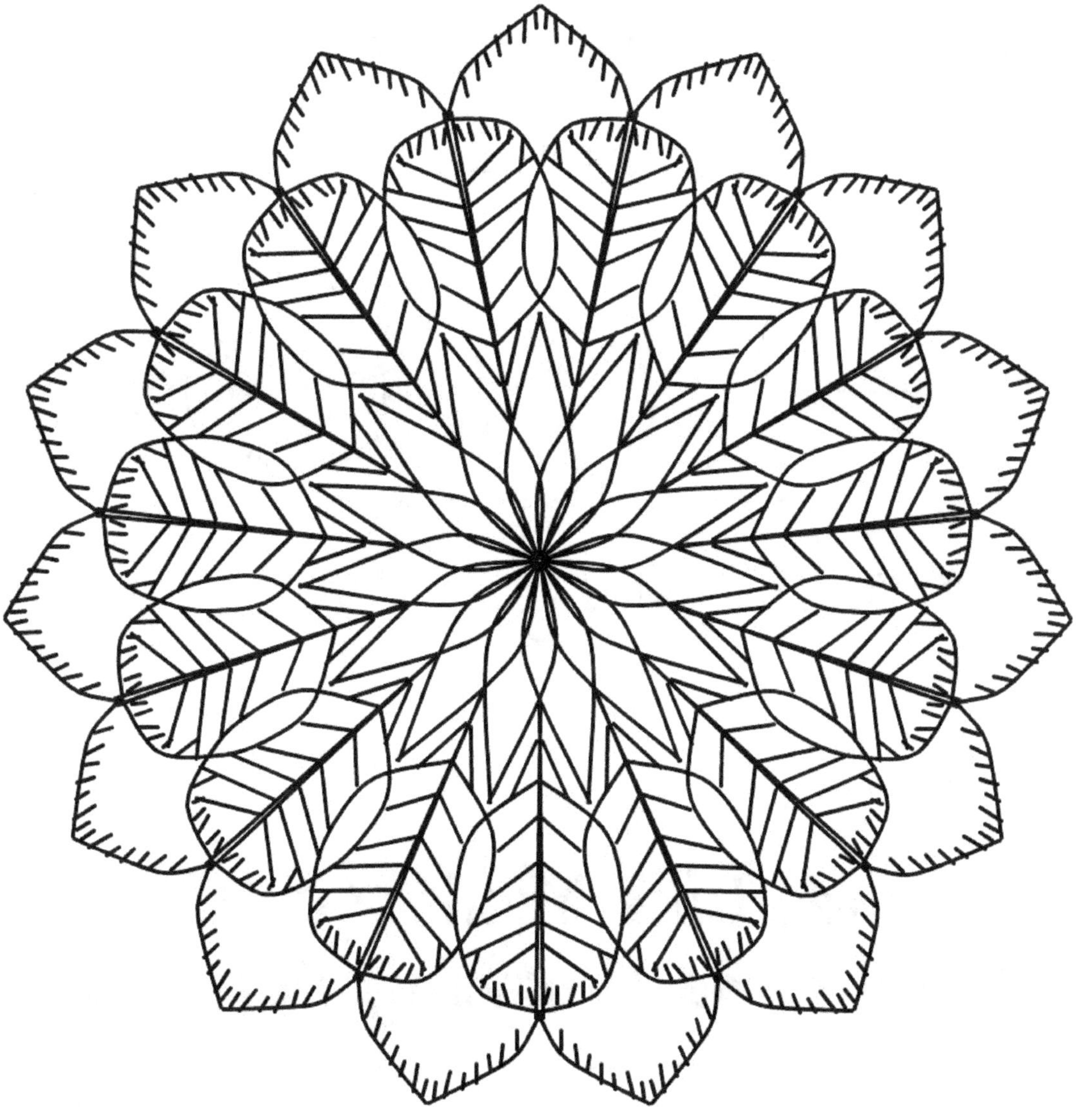

Measurements

P R O G R E S S

DATE: _____________

Weight: _______

Neck _______

Shoulders _______

Chest _______

Bicep / upper arm left _________ right _______

Forearm left _________ right _______

Waist _______

Hips _______

Thighs left _______ right ______

Calf left _________ right _______

C H E C K

Food, Like Your Money,
Should Be Working For You

Day Twenty _________

5:00 _______________________

6:00 _______________________

7:00 _______________________

8:00 _______________________

9:00 _______________________

10:00 ______________________

11:00 ______________________

Noon _______________________

1:00 _______________________

2:00 _______________________

3:00 _______________________

4:00 _______________________

5:00 _______________________

6:00 _______________________

7:00 _______________________

8:00 _______________________

9:00 _______________________

10:00 ______________________

11:00 ______________________

Midnight ___________________

____

____

____

____

What is your level of understanding difficult situations?

____

____

____

____

____

____

The Stella Society Workout

Exercise	Set 1	Set 2	Set 3	Set 4	Set 5	notes

Time started: _____________   Time ended: _______________

Location: ____

Feelings before training: 🙂 😐 ☹️ 😝 😠 😧 😊 😎

Feelings after training 🙂 😐 ☹️ 😝 😠 😧 😊 😎

NUTRITION

Meal 1
time eaten: _________

Meal 2
time eaten: _________

Meal 3
time eaten: _________

Meal 4
time eaten: _________

Meal 5
time eaten: _________

Hydration

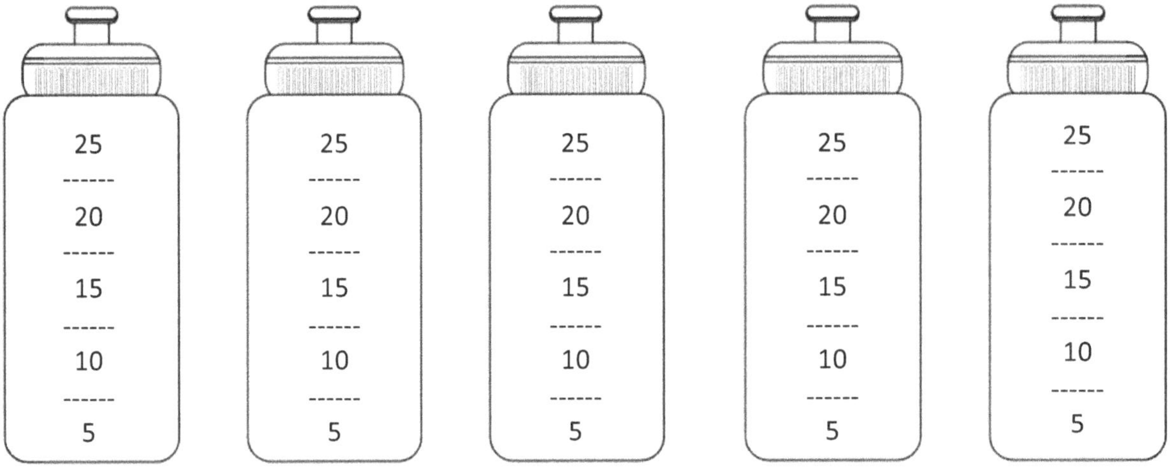

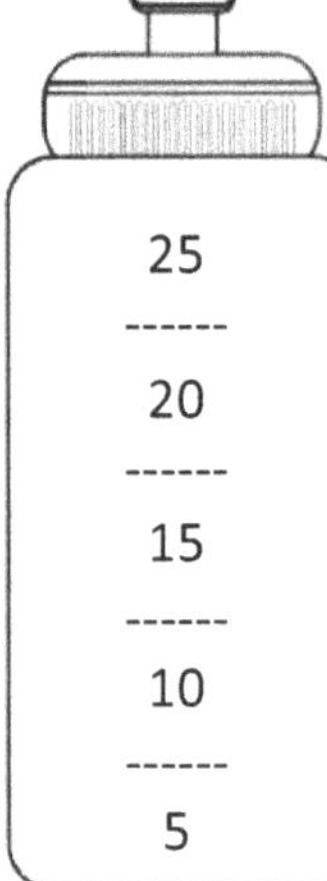

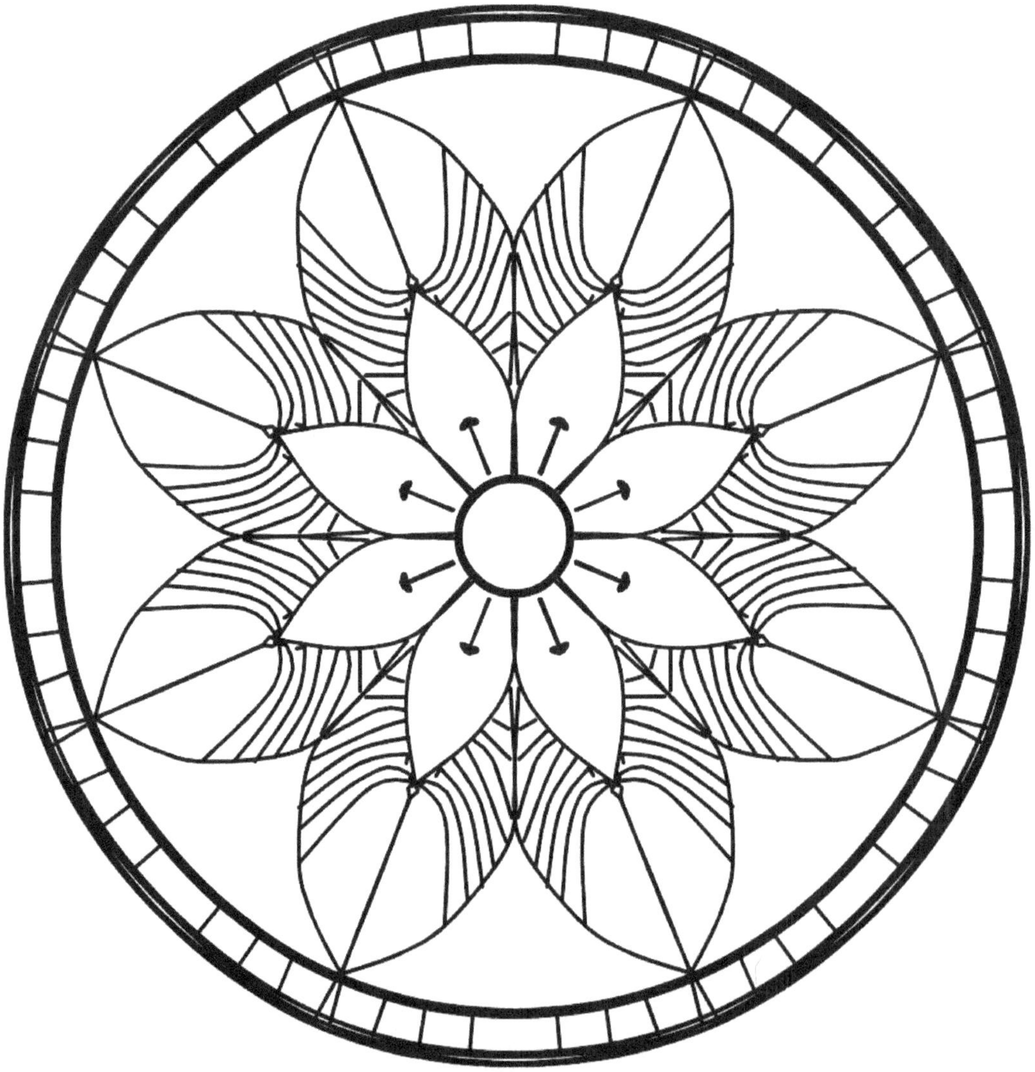

Day Twenty-one ______

5:00 ____________________

6:00 ____________________

7:00 ____________________

8:00 ____________________

9:00 ____________________

10:00 ____________________

11:00 ____________________

Noon ____________________

1:00 ____________________

2:00 ____________________

3:00 ____________________

4:00 ____________________

5:00 ____________________

6:00 ____________________

7:00 ____________________

8:00 ____________________

9:00 ____________________

10:00 ____________________

11:00 ____________________

Midnight ____________________

top priorities for today

____

____

____

____

Today's victories

How much can you endure?

____

____

____

____

____

____

The Stella Society Workout

Exercise	Set 1	Set 2	Set 3	Set 4	Set 5	notes

Time started: _____________ Time ended: _____________

Location: ____

Feelings before training:

Feelings after training

NUTRITION

Meal 1

time eaten: _________

Meal 2

time eaten: _________

Meal 3

time eaten: _________

Meal 4

time eaten: _________

Meal 5

time eaten: _________

Hydration

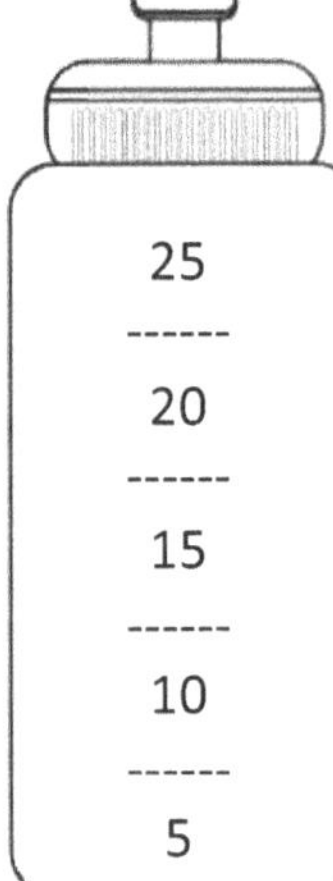

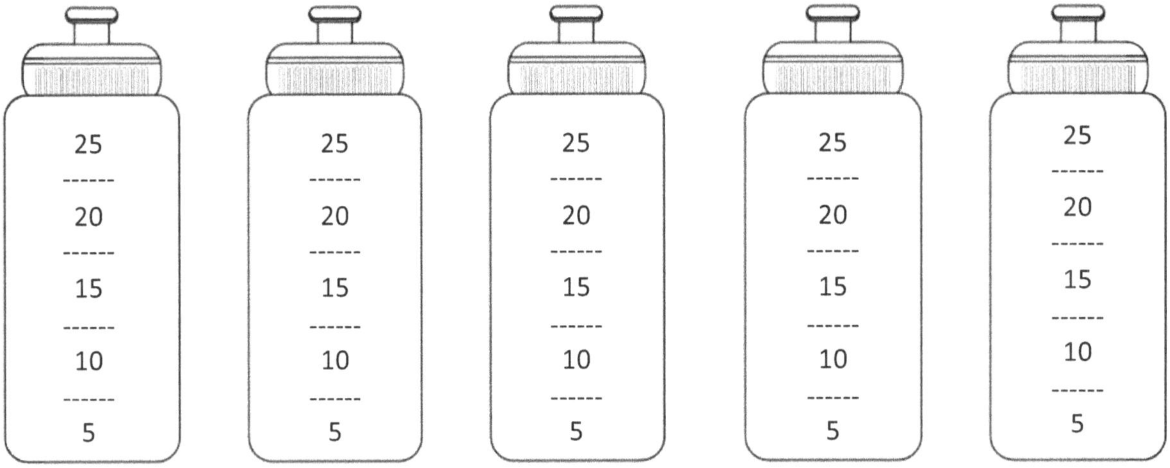

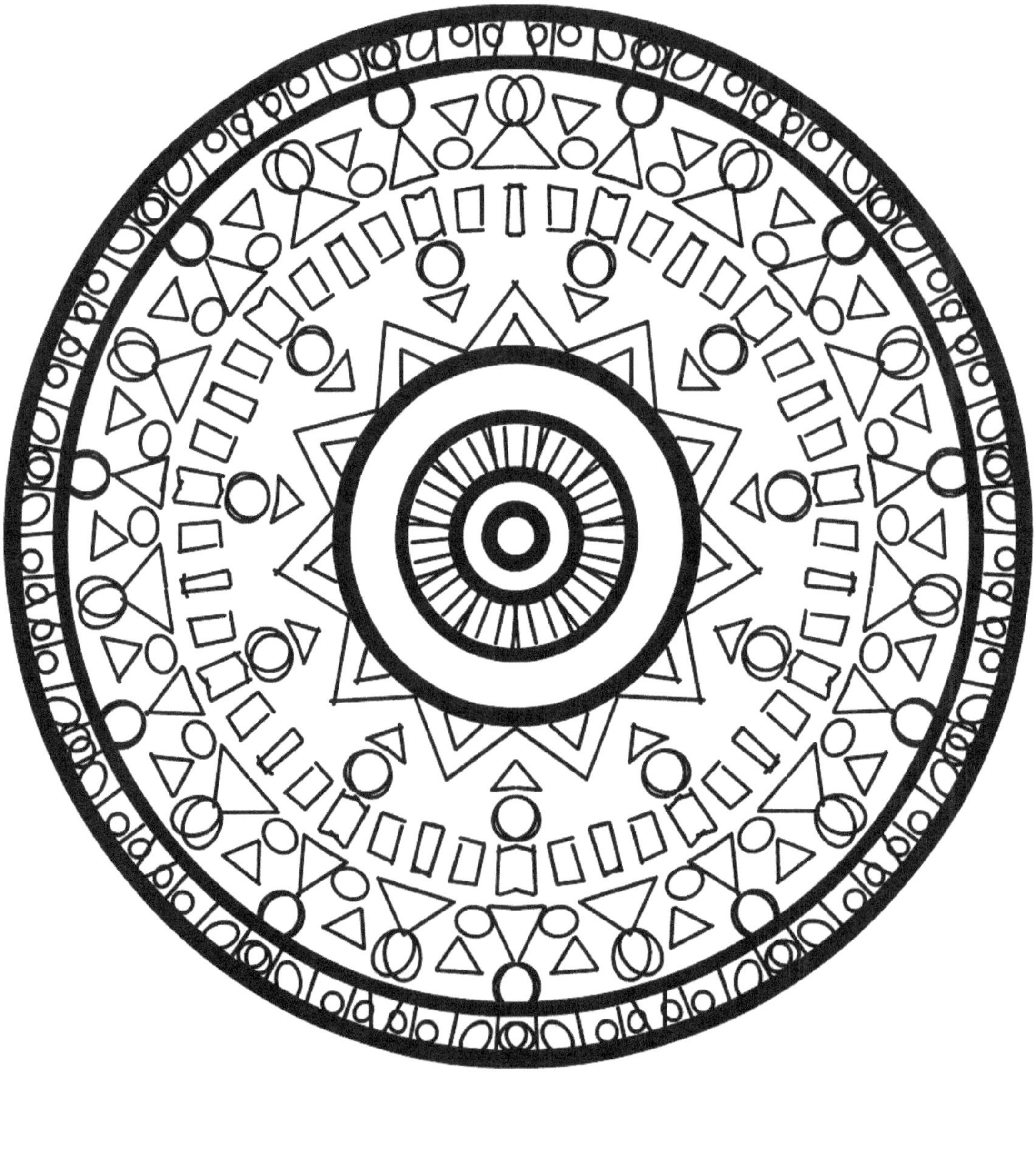

Day Twenty-two _______

5:00 _______________________

6:00 _______________________

7:00 _______________________

8:00 _______________________

9:00 _______________________

10:00 ______________________

11:00 ______________________

Noon _______________________

1:00 _______________________

2:00 _______________________

3:00 _______________________

4:00 _______________________

5:00 _______________________

6:00 _______________________

7:00 _______________________

8:00 _______________________

9:00 _______________________

10:00 ______________________

11:00 ______________________

Midnight ___________________

top priorities for today 🎯

____

____

____

____

Today's victories 🏆

List 5 ways to be thoughtful.

____

____

____

____

____

____

The Stella Society Workout

Exercise	Set 1	Set 2	Set 3	Set 4	Set 5	notes

Time started: _____________ Time ended: _______________

Location: ____

Feelings before training: 🙂 😐 🙁 😜 😣 😦 😊 😎

Feelings after training 🙂 😐 🙁 😜 😣 😦 😊 😎

NUTRITION

Meal 1
time eaten: _________

Meal 2
time eaten: _________

Meal 3
time eaten: _________

Meal 4
time eaten: _________

Meal 5
time eaten: _________

Hydration

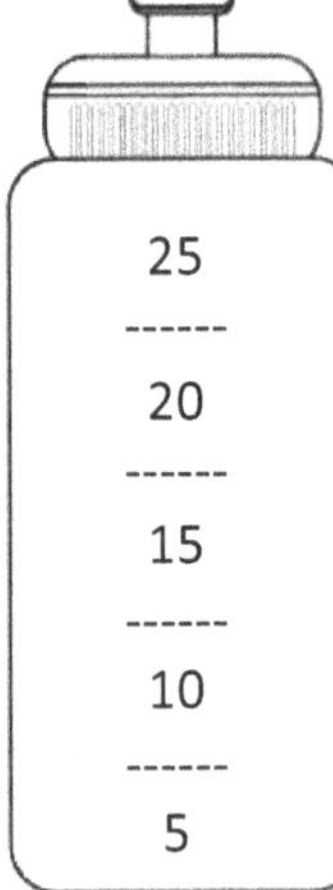

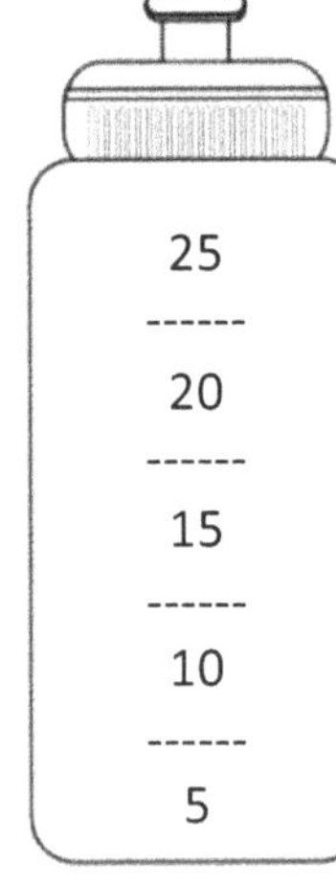

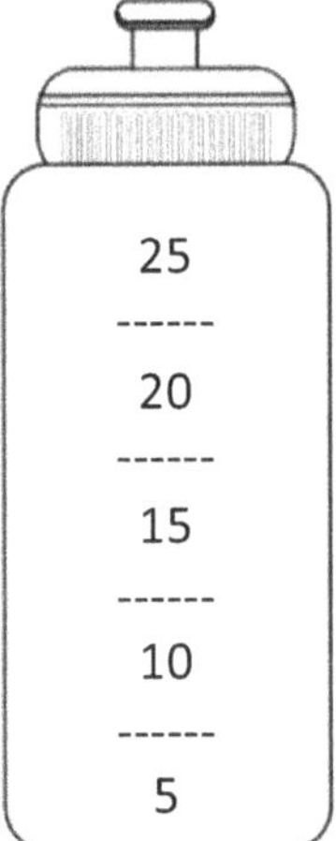

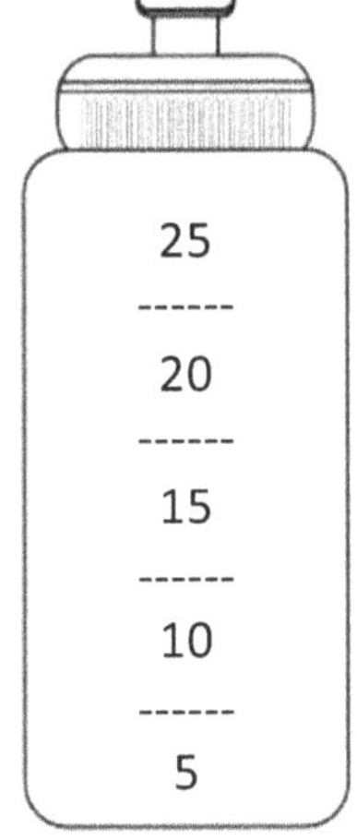

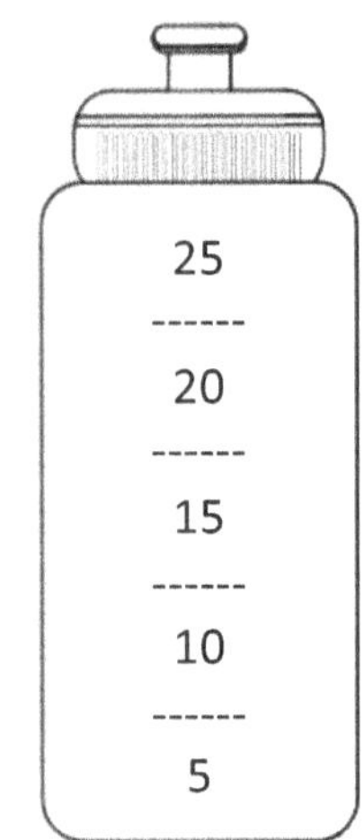

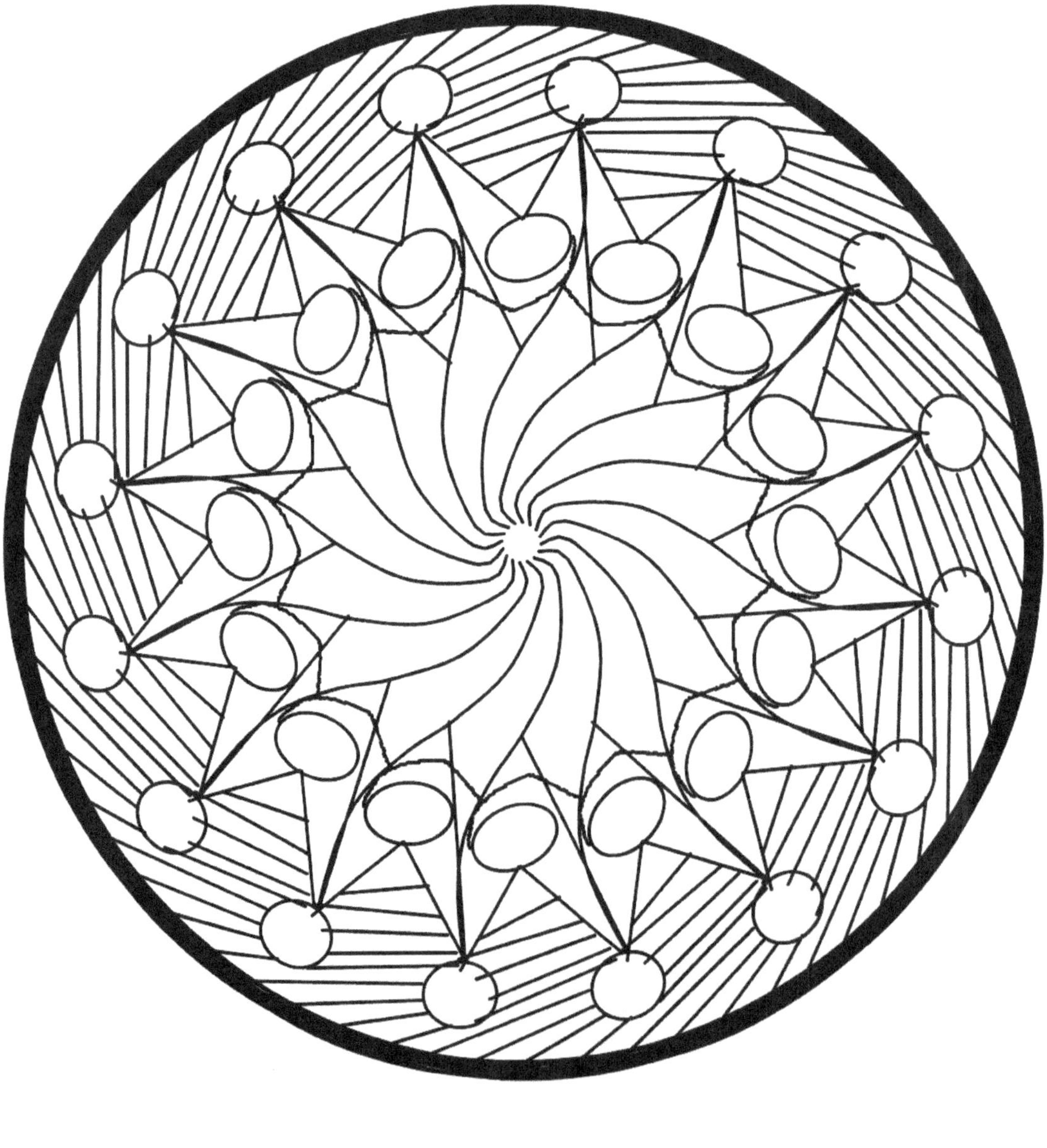

Day Twenty-three _______

5:00 _______________________

6:00 _______________________

7:00 _______________________

8:00 _______________________

9:00 _______________________

10:00 ______________________

11:00 ______________________

Noon _______________________

1:00 _______________________

2:00 _______________________

3:00 _______________________

4:00 _______________________

5:00 _______________________

6:00 _______________________

7:00 _______________________

8:00 _______________________

9:00 _______________________

10:00 ______________________

11:00 ______________________

Midnight ___________________

____

____

____

____

Why should you be unapologetic?

____

____

____

____

____

____

The Stella Society Workout

Exercise	Set 1	Set 2	Set 3	Set 4	Set 5	notes

Time started: ______________   Time ended: ________________

Location: ____

Feelings before training:

Feelings after training

NUTRITION

Meal 1

time eaten: _________

Meal 2

time eaten: _________

Meal 3

time eaten: _________

Meal 4

time eaten: _________

Meal 5

time eaten: _________

Hydration

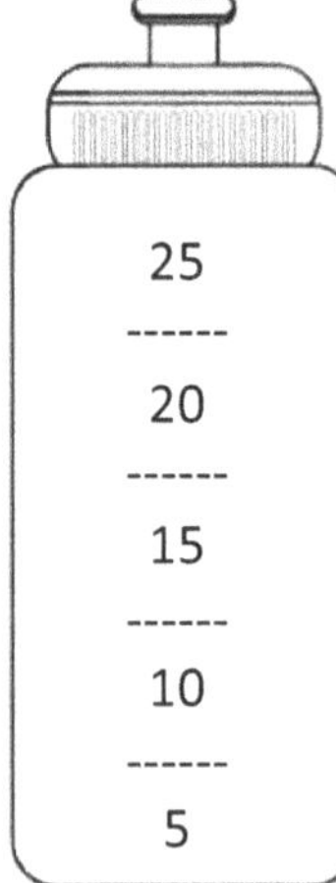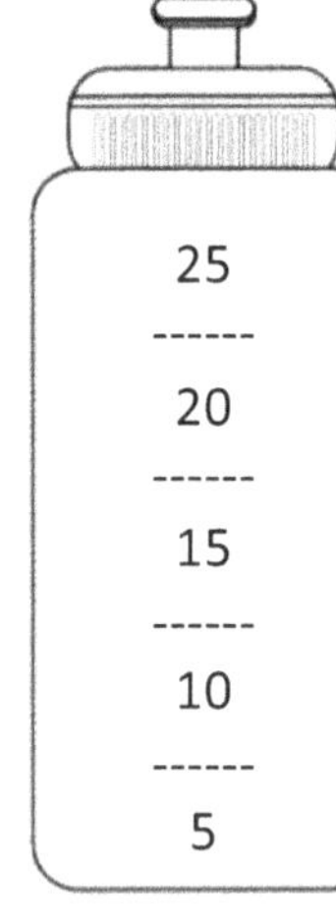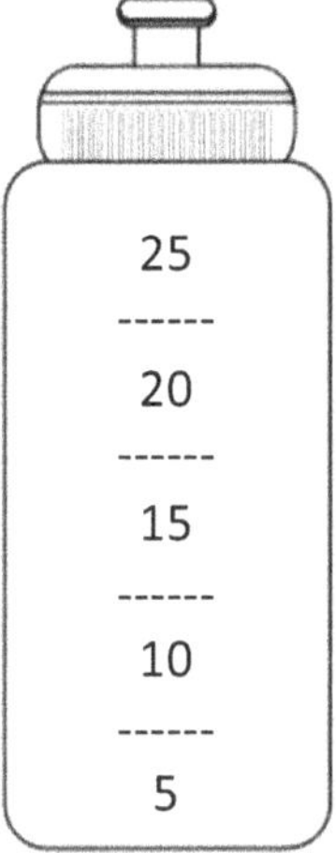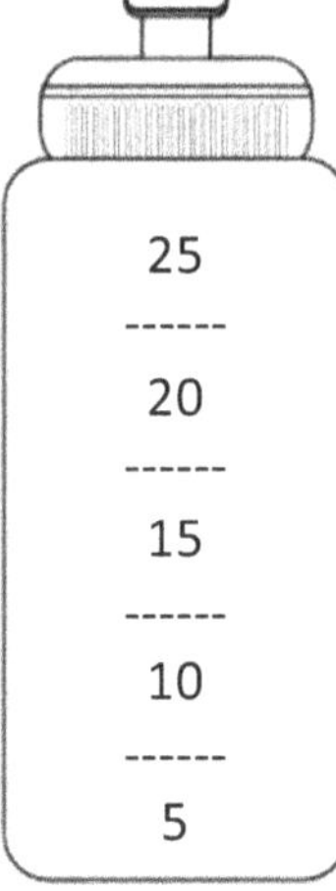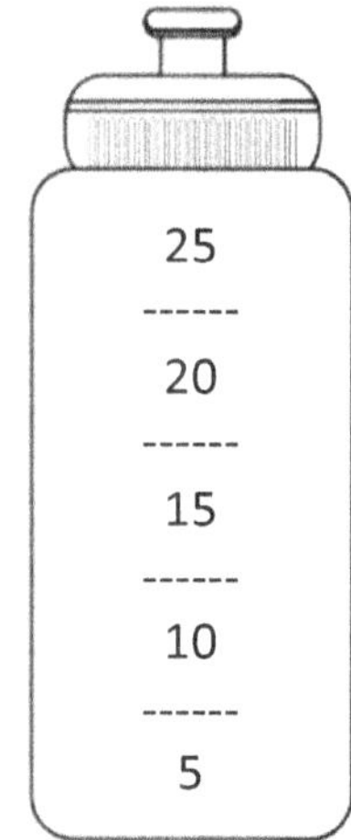

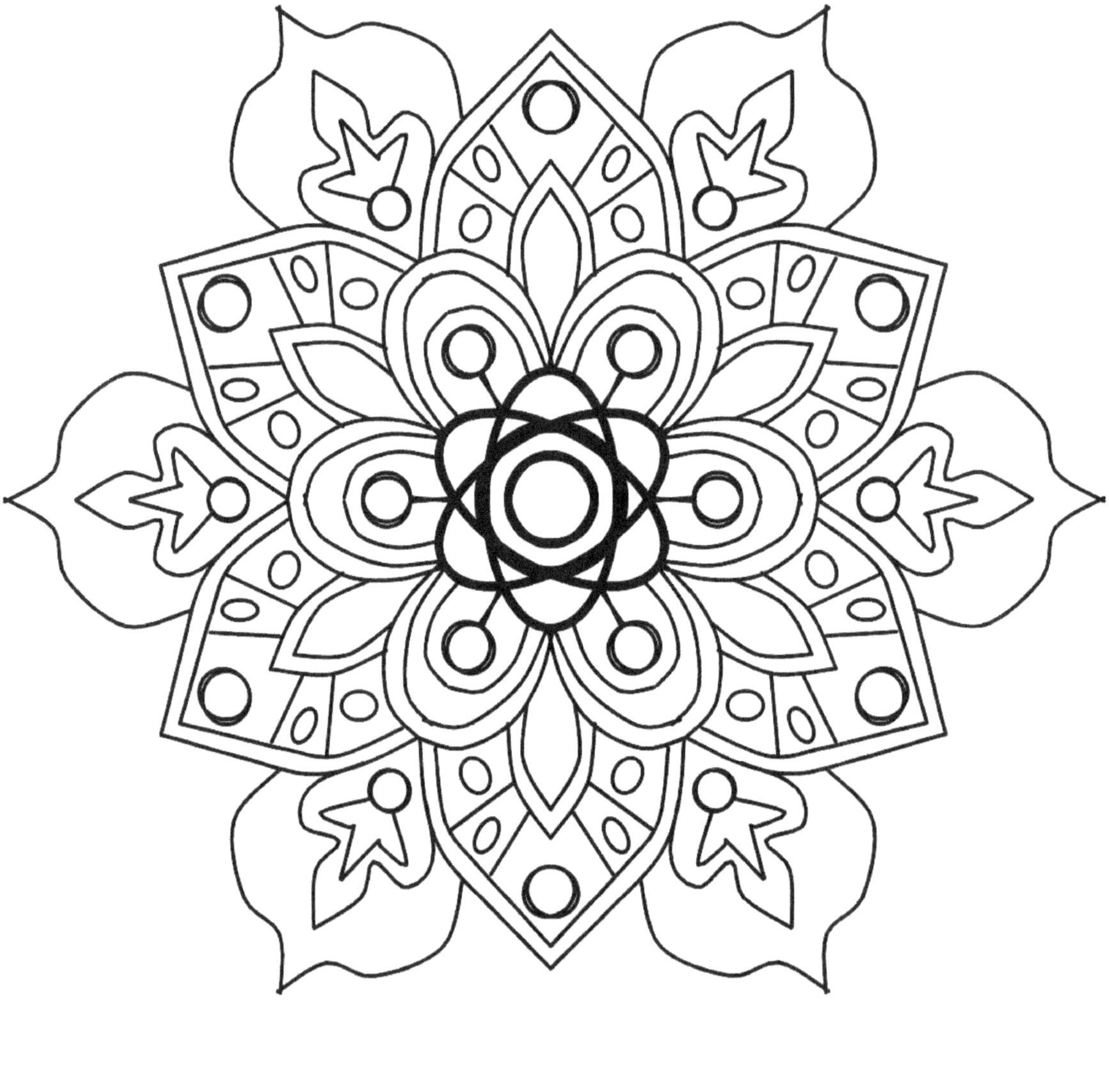

Day Twenty-four _______

top priorities for today

Today's victories

What can you set on fire
with your fierceness?

The Stella Society Workout

Exercise	Set 1	Set 2	Set 3	Set 4	Set 5	notes

Time started: _____________ Time ended: _____________

Location: ____

Feelings before training:

Feelings after training

NUTRITION

Meal 1
time eaten: _________

Meal 2
time eaten: _________

Meal 3
time eaten: _________

Meal 4
time eaten: _________

Meal 5
time eaten: _________

Hydration

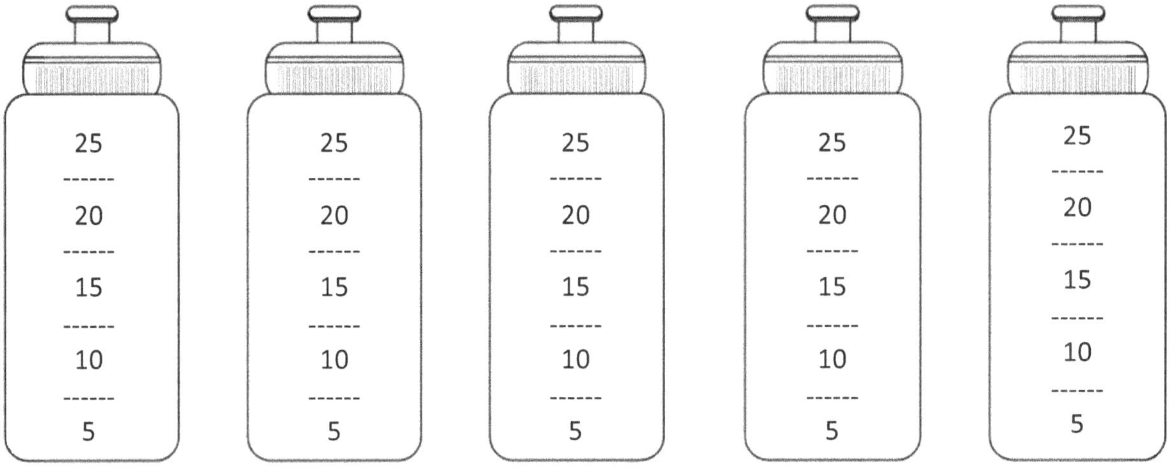

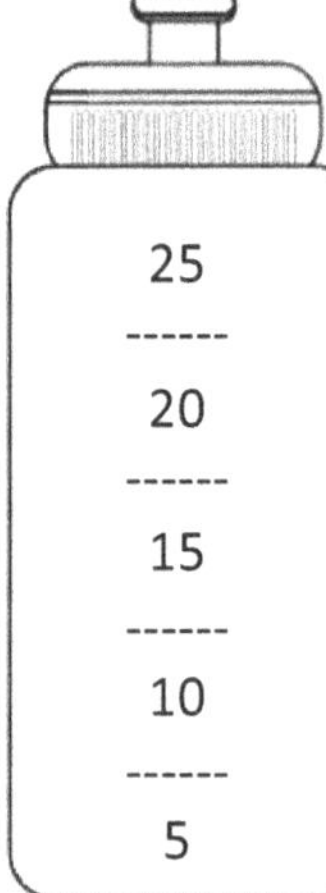

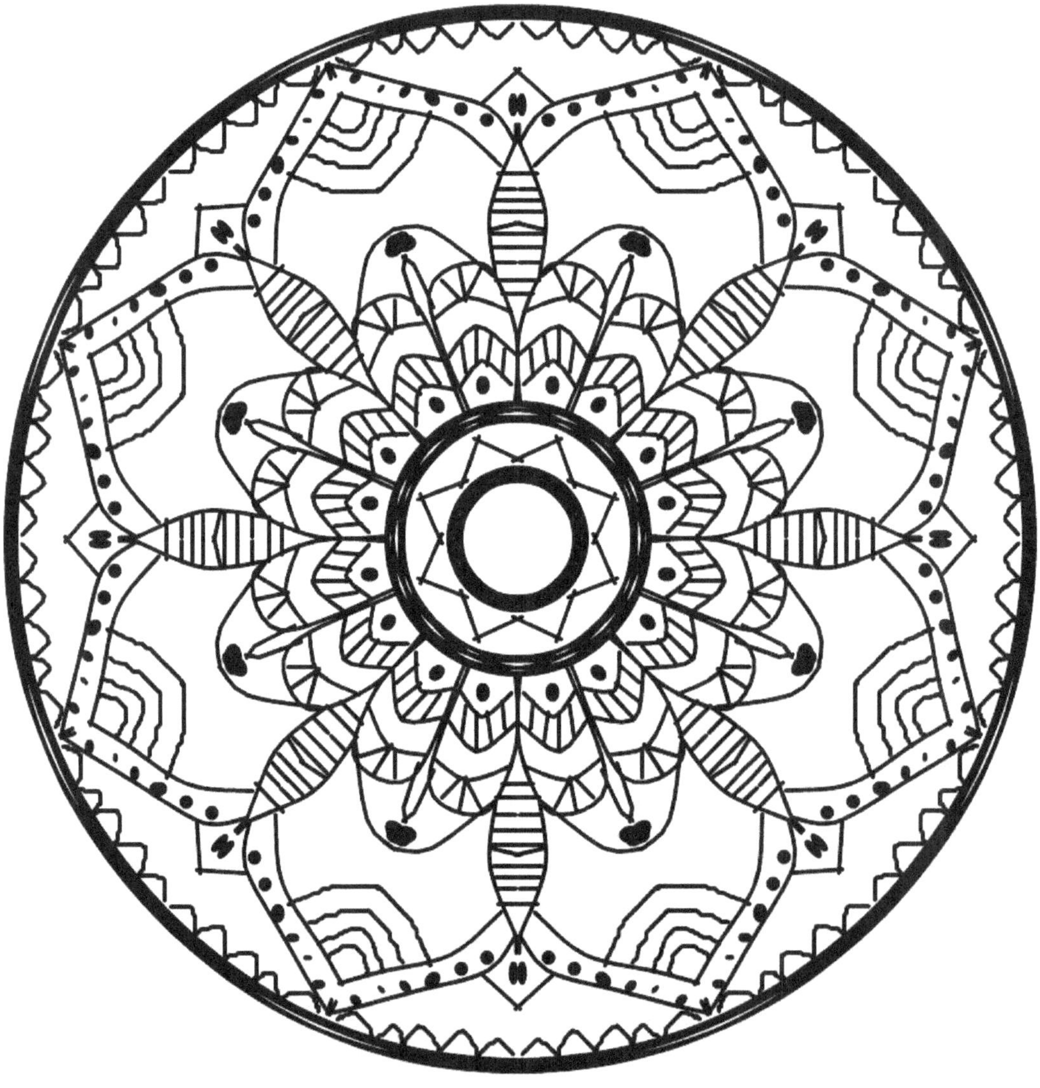

Day Twenty-five ______

5:00 ______________________

6:00 ______________________

7:00 ______________________

8:00 ______________________

9:00 ______________________

10:00 ____________________

11:00 ____________________

Noon _____________________

1:00 ______________________

2:00 ______________________

3:00 ______________________

4:00 ______________________

5:00 ______________________

6:00 ______________________

7:00 ______________________

8:00 ______________________

9:00 ______________________

10:00 ____________________

11:00 ____________________

Midnight _________________

top priorities for today 

____

____

____

____

Today's victories 🏆

Make it your mission to stay positive. Write your positive mission statement.

____

____

____

____

____

The Workout

Exercise	Set 1	Set 2	Set 3	Set 4	Set 5	notes

Time started: _______________   Time ended: _______________

Location: ____

Feelings before training:

Feelings after training

NUTRITION

Meal 1

time eaten: _________

Meal 2

time eaten: _________

Meal 3

time eaten: _________

Meal 4

time eaten: _________

Meal 5

time eaten: _________

Hydration

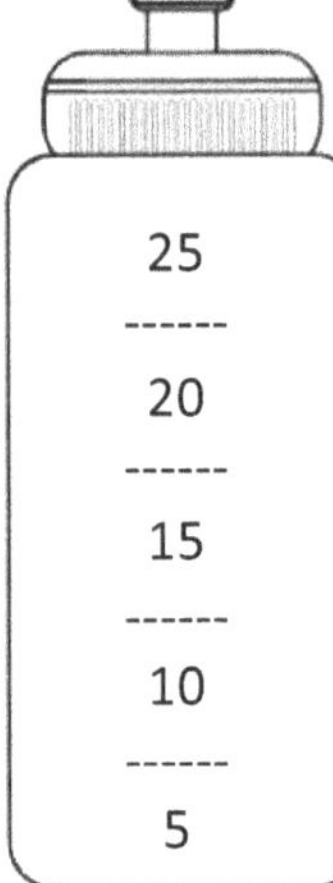 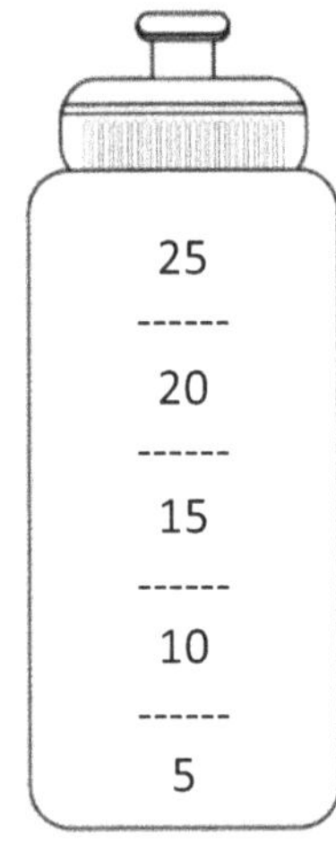 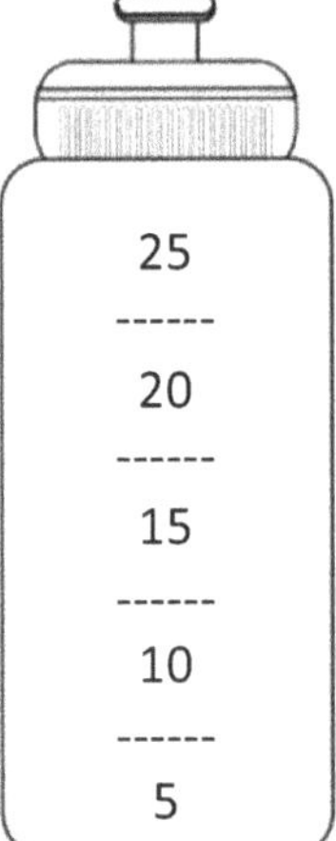 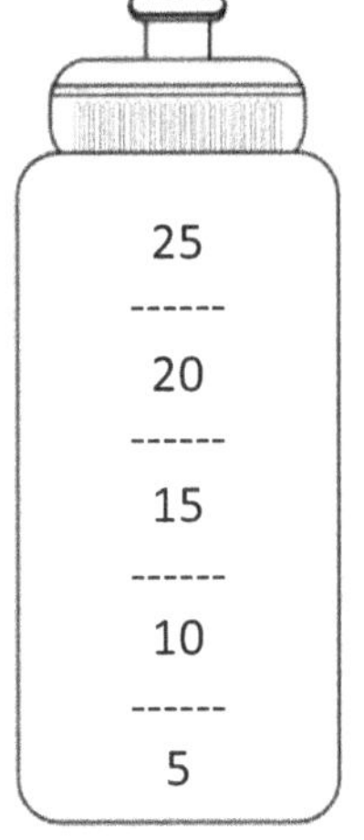 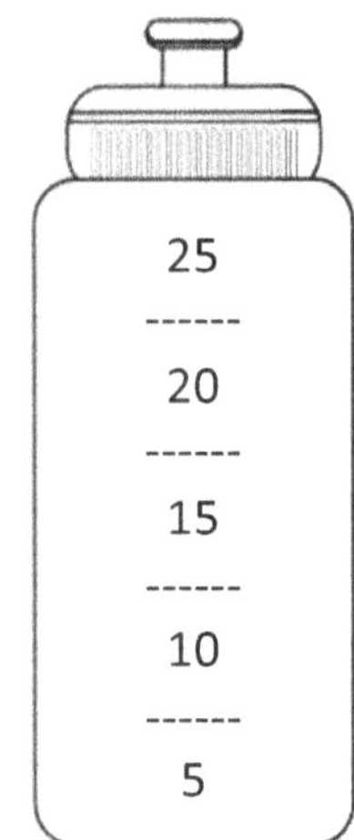

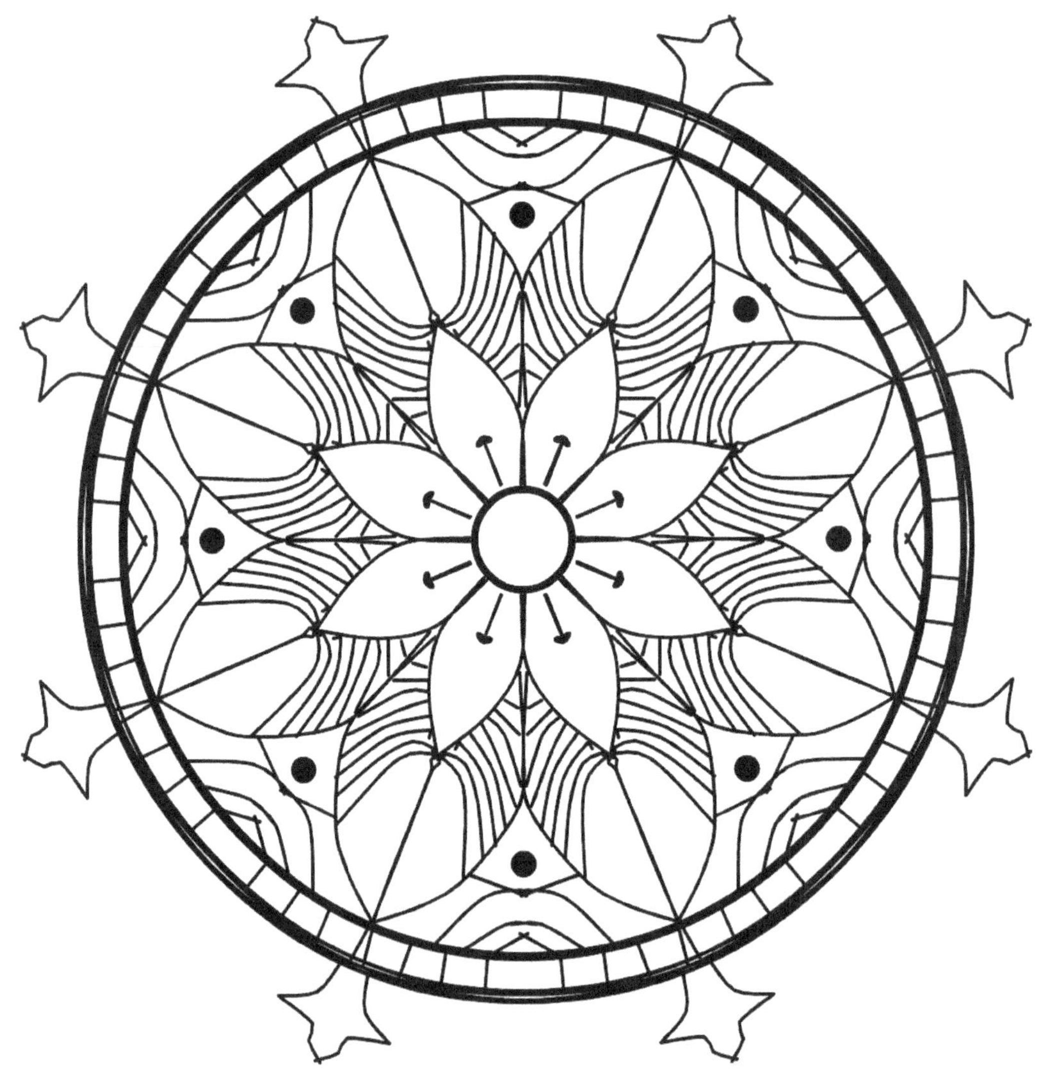

Day Twenty-six _______

5:00 ______________________

6:00 ______________________

7:00 ______________________

8:00 ______________________

9:00 ______________________

10:00 ____________________

11:00 ____________________

Noon _____________________

1:00 ______________________

2:00 ______________________

3:00 ______________________

4:00 ______________________

5:00 ______________________

6:00 ______________________

7:00 ______________________

8:00 ______________________

9:00 ______________________

10:00 ____________________

11:00 ____________________

Midnight _________________

top priorities for today

Today's victories

What give you your inner energy?

The Workout

Exercise	Set 1	Set 2	Set 3	Set 4	Set 5	notes

Time started: ________________ Time ended: ________________

Location: ____

Feelings before training:

Feelings after training

NUTRITION

Meal 1

time eaten: _________

Meal 2

time eaten: _________

Meal 3

time eaten: _________

Meal 4

time eaten: _________

Meal 5

time eaten: _________

Hydration

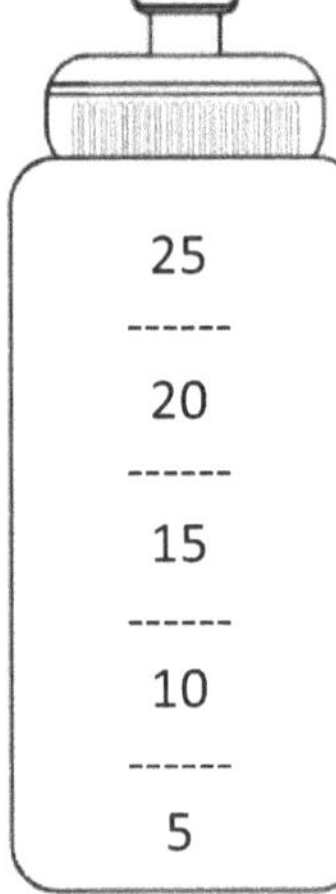
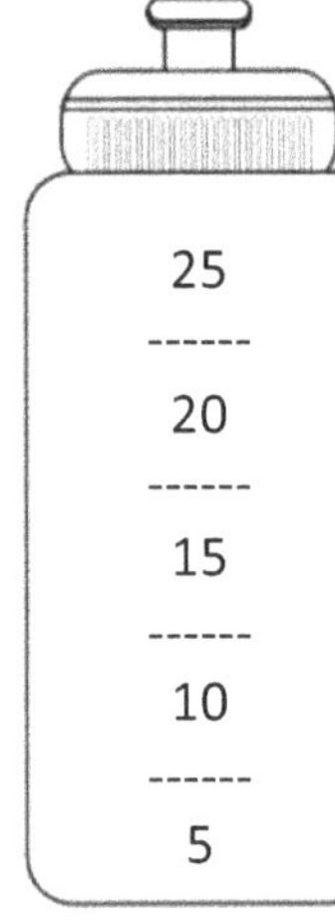
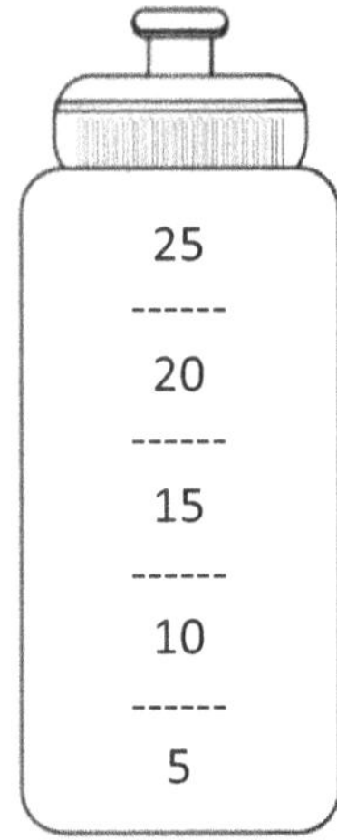

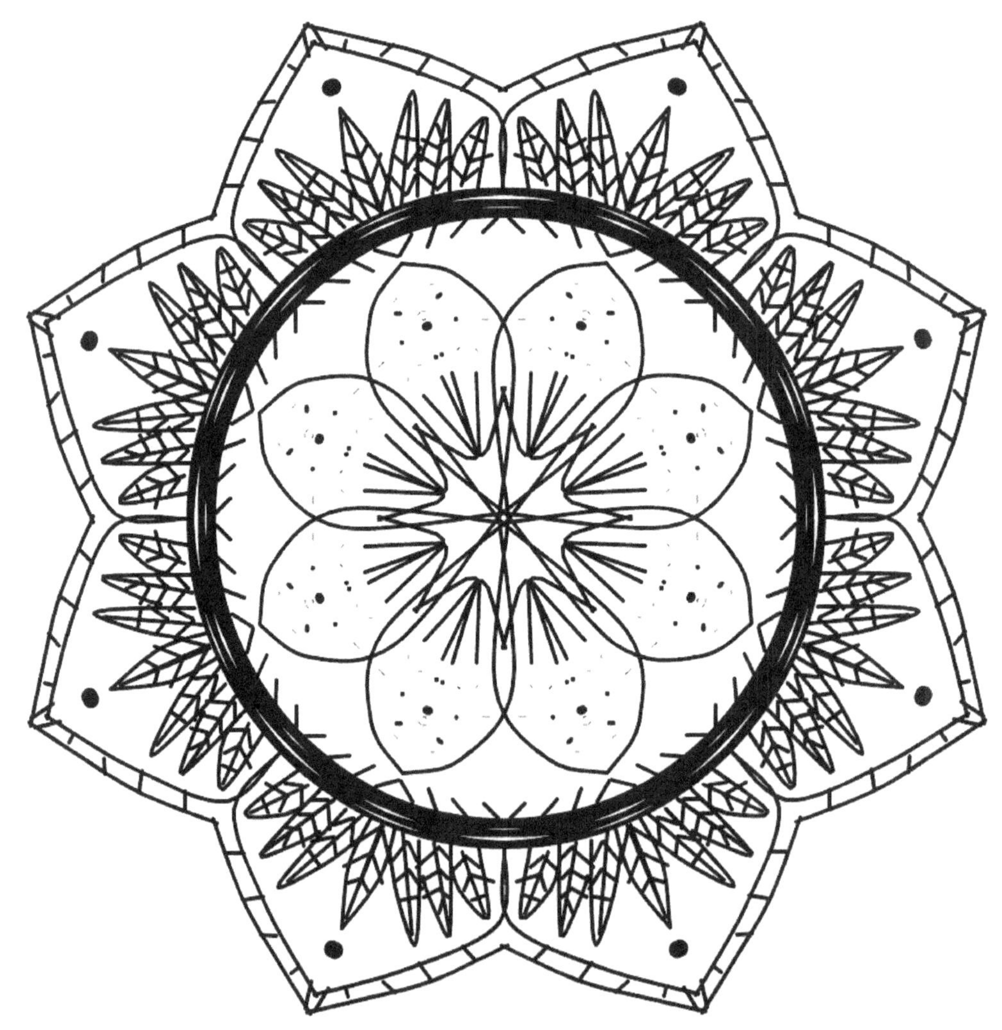

Day Twenty-seven _______

5:00 _______________________

6:00 _______________________

7:00 _______________________

8:00 _______________________

9:00 _______________________

10:00 _______________________

11:00 _______________________

Noon _______________________

1:00 _______________________

2:00 _______________________

3:00 _______________________

4:00 _______________________

5:00 _______________________

6:00 _______________________

7:00 _______________________

8:00 _______________________

9:00 _______________________

10:00 _______________________

11:00 _______________________

Midnight _______________________

____

____

____

____

____

What have you stopped, but won't stop again?

____

____

____

____

____

____

The Workout

Exercise	Set 1	Set 2	Set 3	Set 4	Set 5	notes

Time started: _____________   Time ended: _______________

Location: ____

Feelings before training: 🙂 😐 🙁 😜 😠 😒 😊 😎

Feelings after training 🙂 😐 🙁 😜 😠 😒 😊 😎

NUTRITION

Meal 1
time eaten: _________

Meal 2
time eaten: _________

Meal 3
time eaten: _________

Meal 4
time eaten: _________

Meal 5
time eaten: _________

Hydration

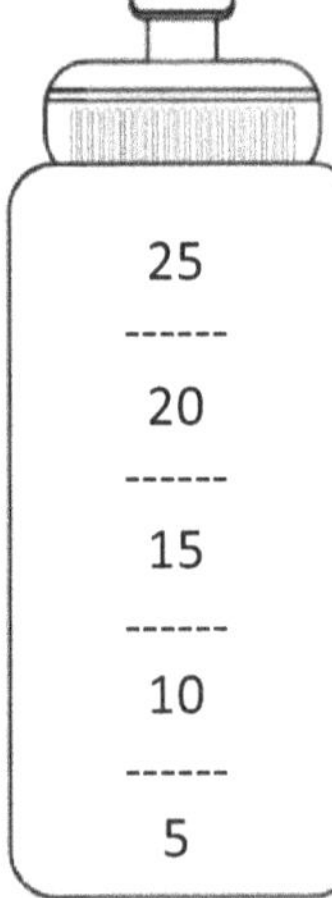

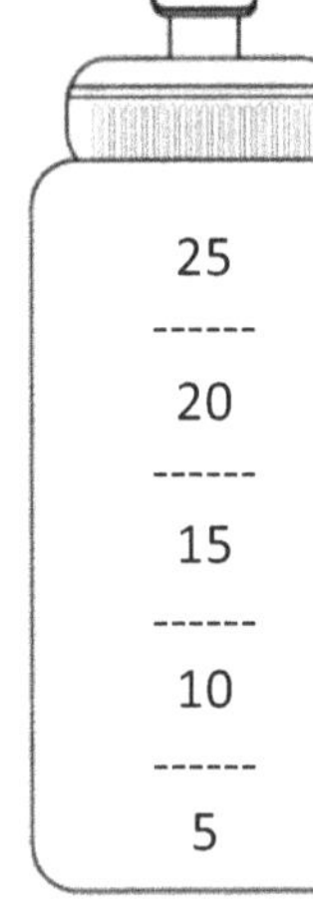

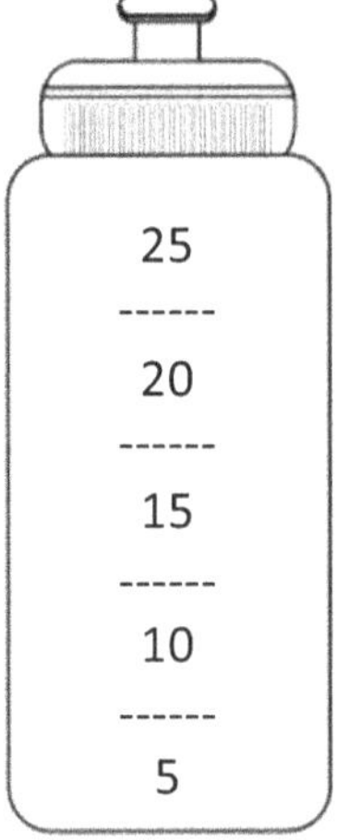

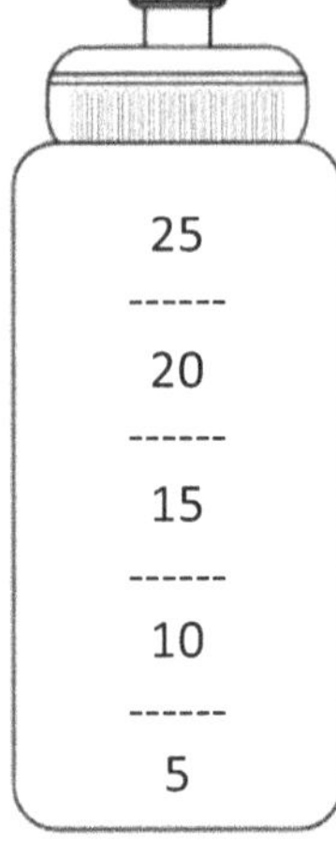

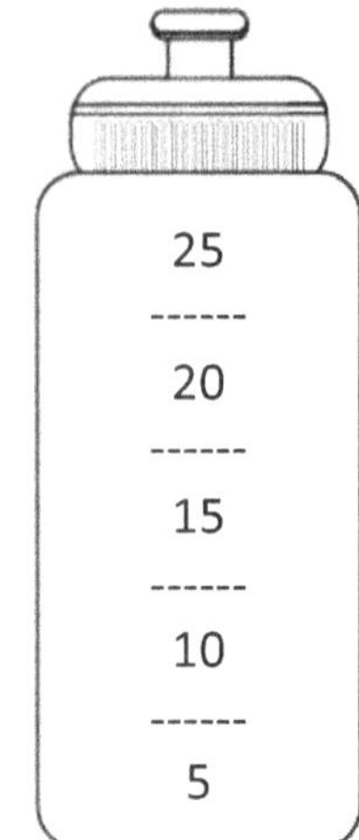

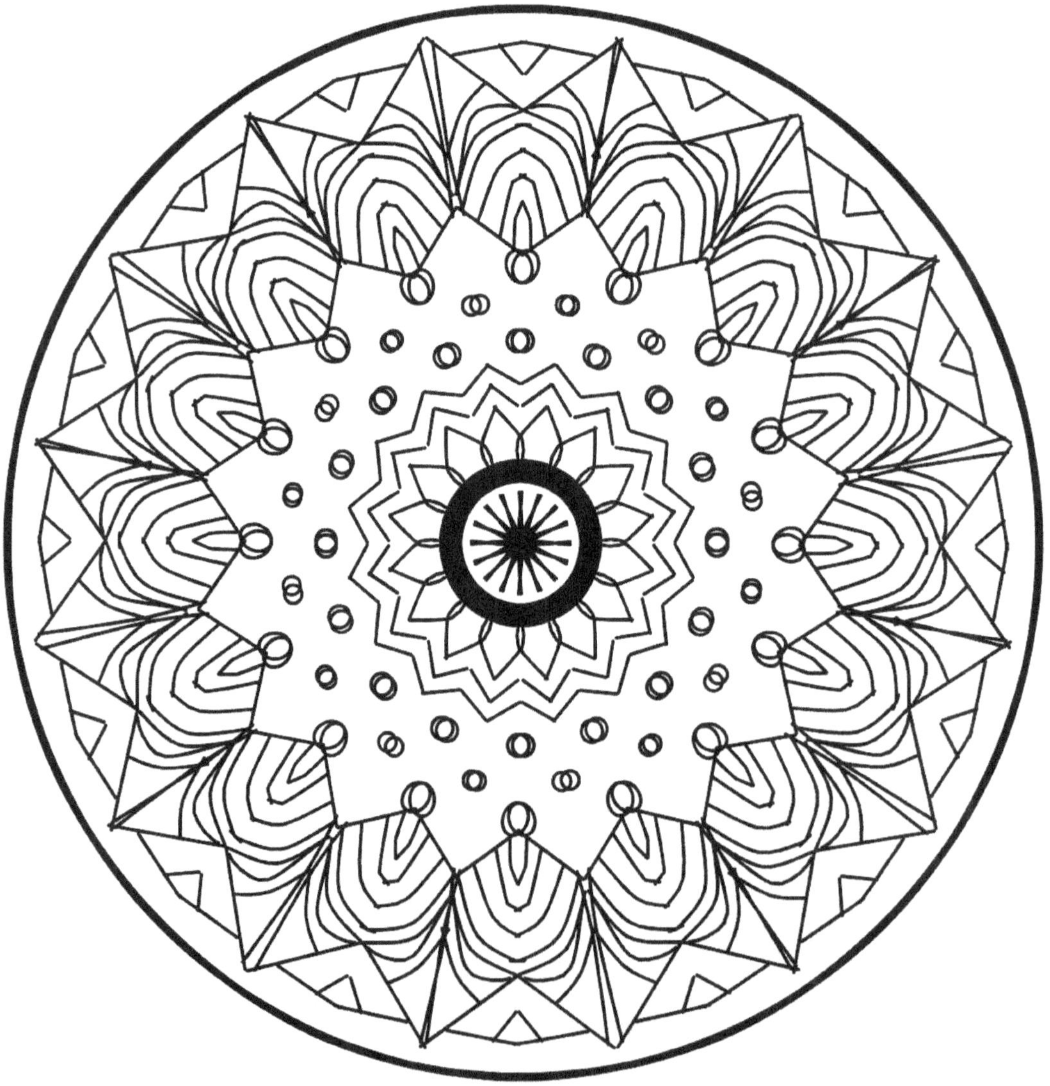

Day Twenty-eight _______

5:00 _________________________

6:00 _________________________

7:00 _________________________

8:00 _________________________

9:00 _________________________

10:00 ________________________

11:00 ________________________

Noon _________________________

1:00 _________________________

2:00 _________________________

3:00 _________________________

4:00 _________________________

5:00 _________________________

6:00 _________________________

7:00 _________________________

8:00 _________________________

9:00 _________________________

10:00 ________________________

11:00 ________________________

Midnight _____________________

top priorities for today

____

____

____

____

____

Today's victories

How do identify with being a unicorn?

____

____

____

____

____

____

____

The Stella Society Workout

Exercise	Set 1	Set 2	Set 3	Set 4	Set 5	notes

Time started: _______________ Time ended: _______________

Location: ____

Feelings before training:

Feelings after training

NUTRITION

Meal 1

time eaten: _________

Meal 2

time eaten: _________

Meal 3

time eaten: _________

Meal 4

time eaten: _________

Meal 5

time eaten: _________

Hydration

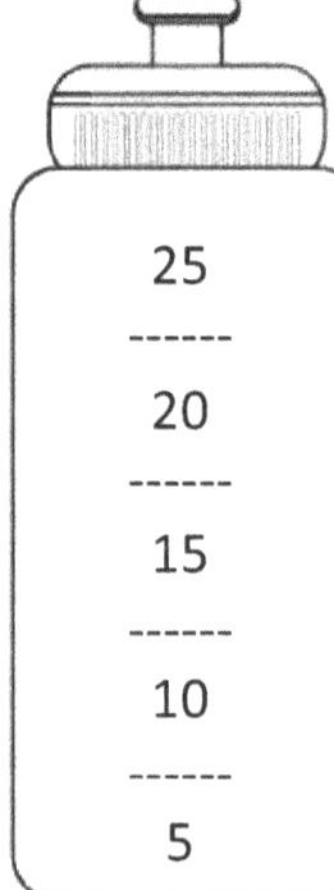

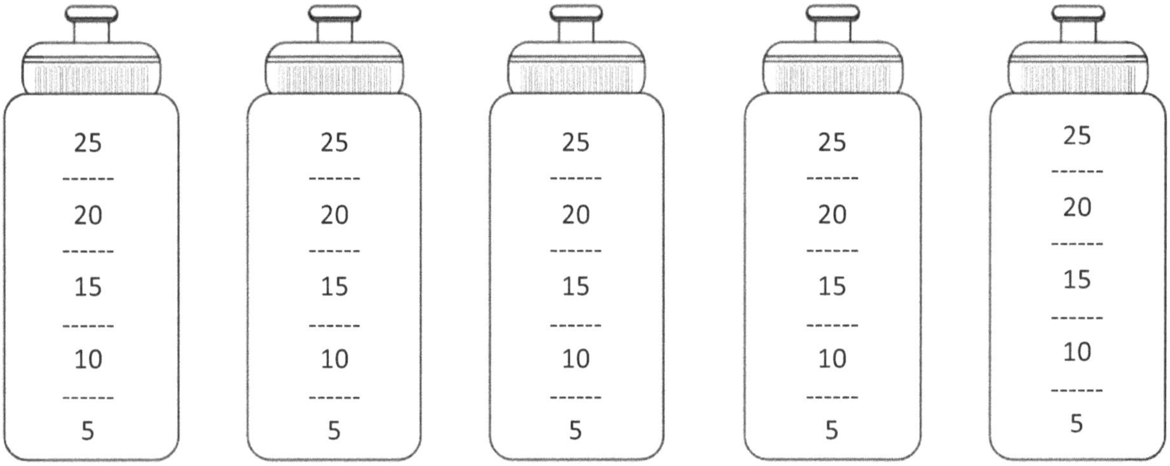

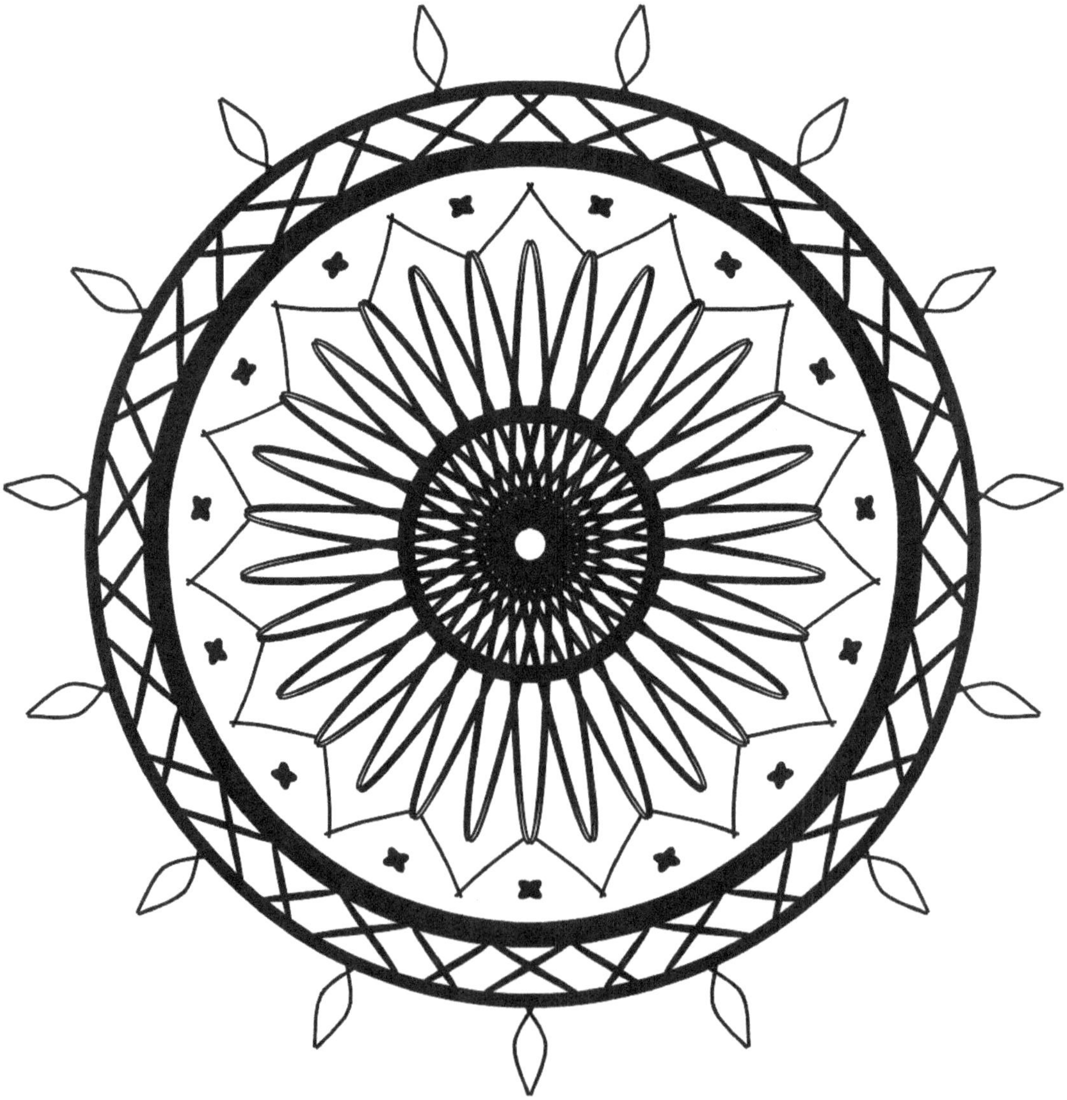

Day Twenty-nine _______

5:00 ____________________	

5:00 _______________________

6:00 _______________________

7:00 _______________________

8:00 _______________________

9:00 _______________________

10:00 ______________________

11:00 ______________________

Noon _______________________

1:00 _______________________

2:00 _______________________

3:00 _______________________

4:00 _______________________

5:00 _______________________

6:00 _______________________

7:00 _______________________

8:00 _______________________

9:00 _______________________

10:00 ______________________

11:00 ______________________

Midnight __________________

top priorities for today 🎯

____

____

____

____

Today's victories 🏆

You have permission to be a savage. What do you do with it?

____

____

____

____

____

____

The Stella Society Workout

Exercise	Set 1	Set 2	Set 3	Set 4	Set 5	notes

Time started: _____________   Time ended: _______________

Location: ____

Feelings before training: 🙂 😐 🙁 😜 😣 😟 😊 😎

Feelings after training 🙂 😐 🙁 😜 😣 😟 😊 😎

NUTRITION

Meal 1

time eaten: _________

Meal 2

time eaten: _________

Meal 3

time eaten: _________

Meal 4

time eaten: _________

Meal 5

time eaten: _________

Hydration

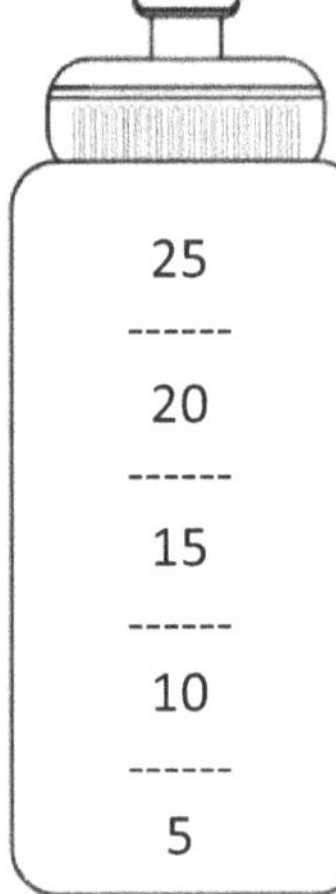

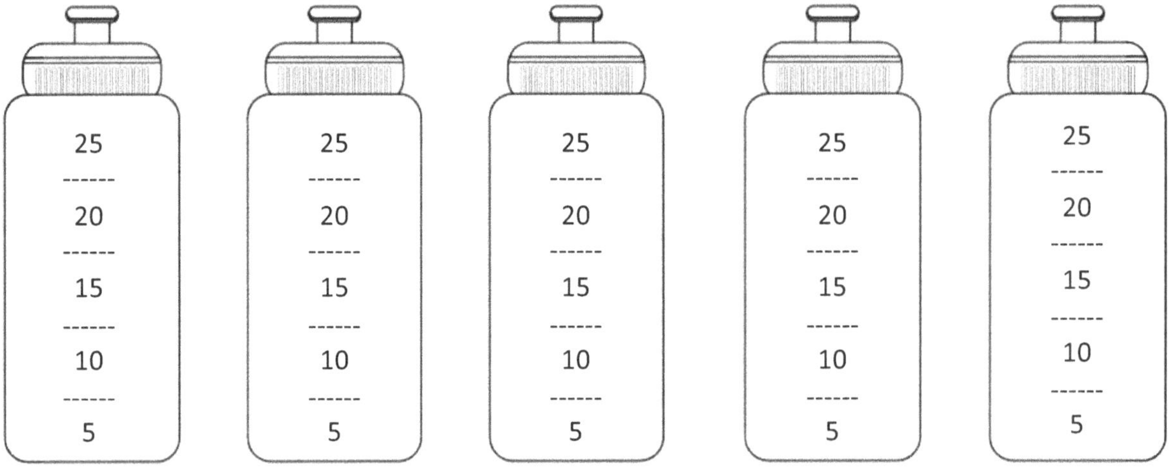

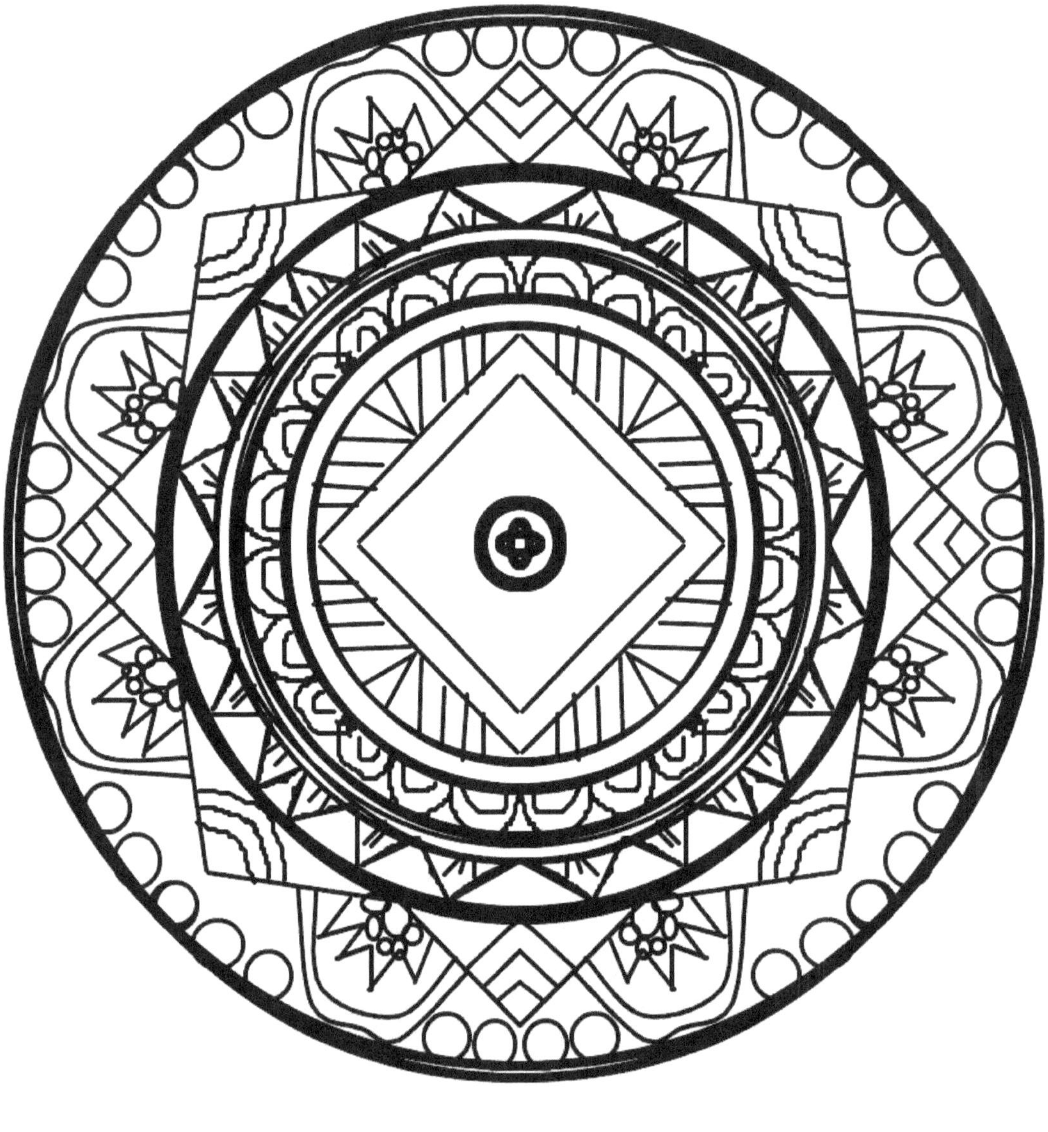

Measurements

DATE: ___________

Weight: _______

Neck _______

Shoulders _______

Chest _______

Bicep / upper arm left _________ right _______

Forearm left _________ right _______

Waist _______

Hips _______

Thighs left _________ right _______

Calf left _________ right _______

It's Not A Diet,
It's A Lifestyle Change

Day Thirty _______

top priorities for today

5:00 _______________________

6:00 _______________________

7:00 _______________________

8:00 _______________________

9:00 _______________________

10:00 _______________________

11:00 _______________________

Noon _______________________

1:00 _______________________

2:00 _______________________

3:00 _______________________

4:00 _______________________

5:00 _______________________

6:00 _______________________

7:00 _______________________

8:00 _______________________

9:00 _______________________

10:00 _______________________

11:00 _______________________

Midnight _______________________

Today's victories

How can you be powerful and sensitive at the same time?

The Stella Society Workout

Exercise	Set 1	Set 2	Set 3	Set 4	Set 5	notes

Time started: _____________ Time ended: _____________

Location: ____

Feelings before training:        

Feelings after training

NUTRITION

Meal 1
time eaten: _________

Meal 2
time eaten: _________

Meal 3
time eaten: _________

Meal 4
time eaten: _________

Meal 5
time eaten: _________

Hydration

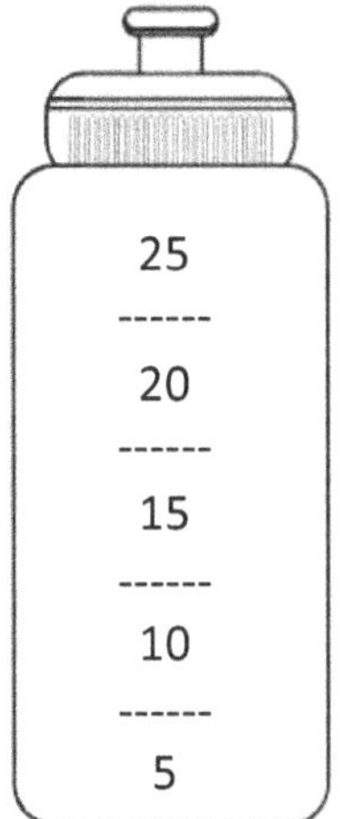
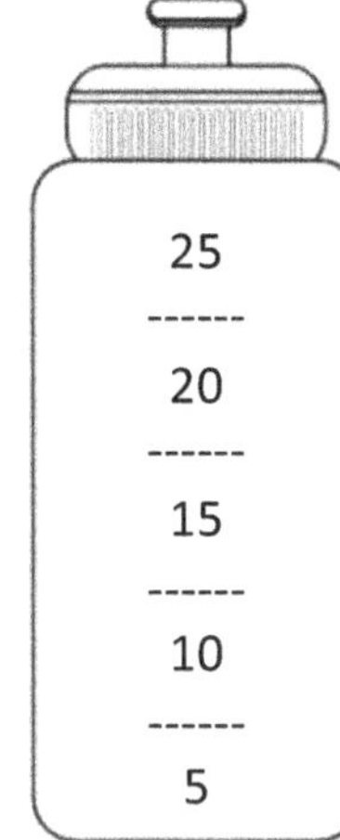
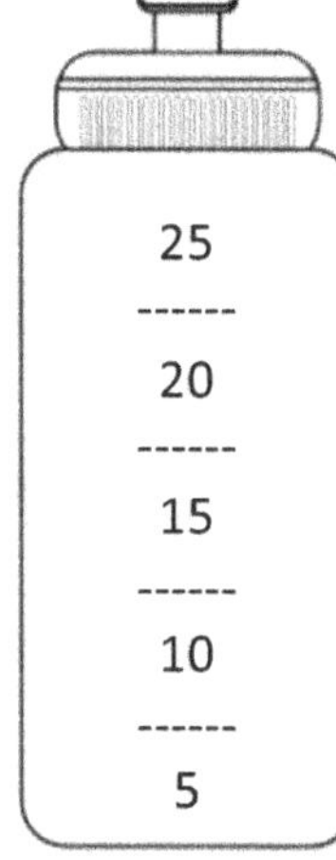
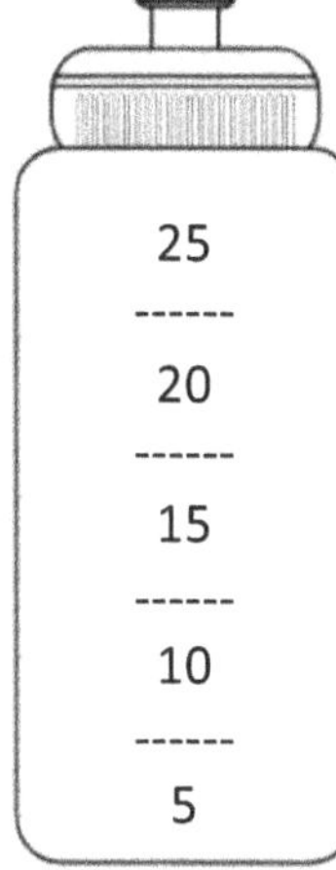
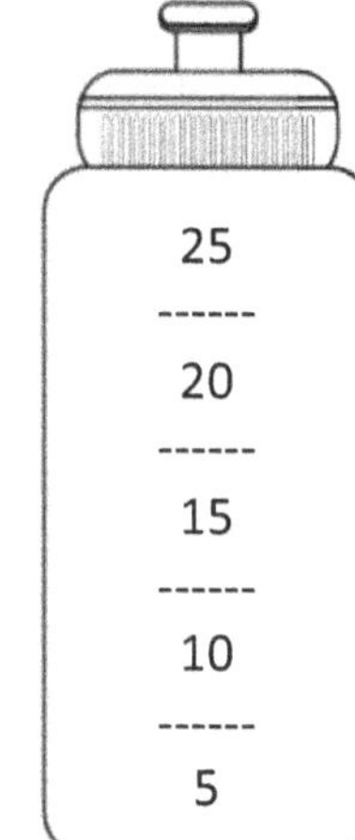

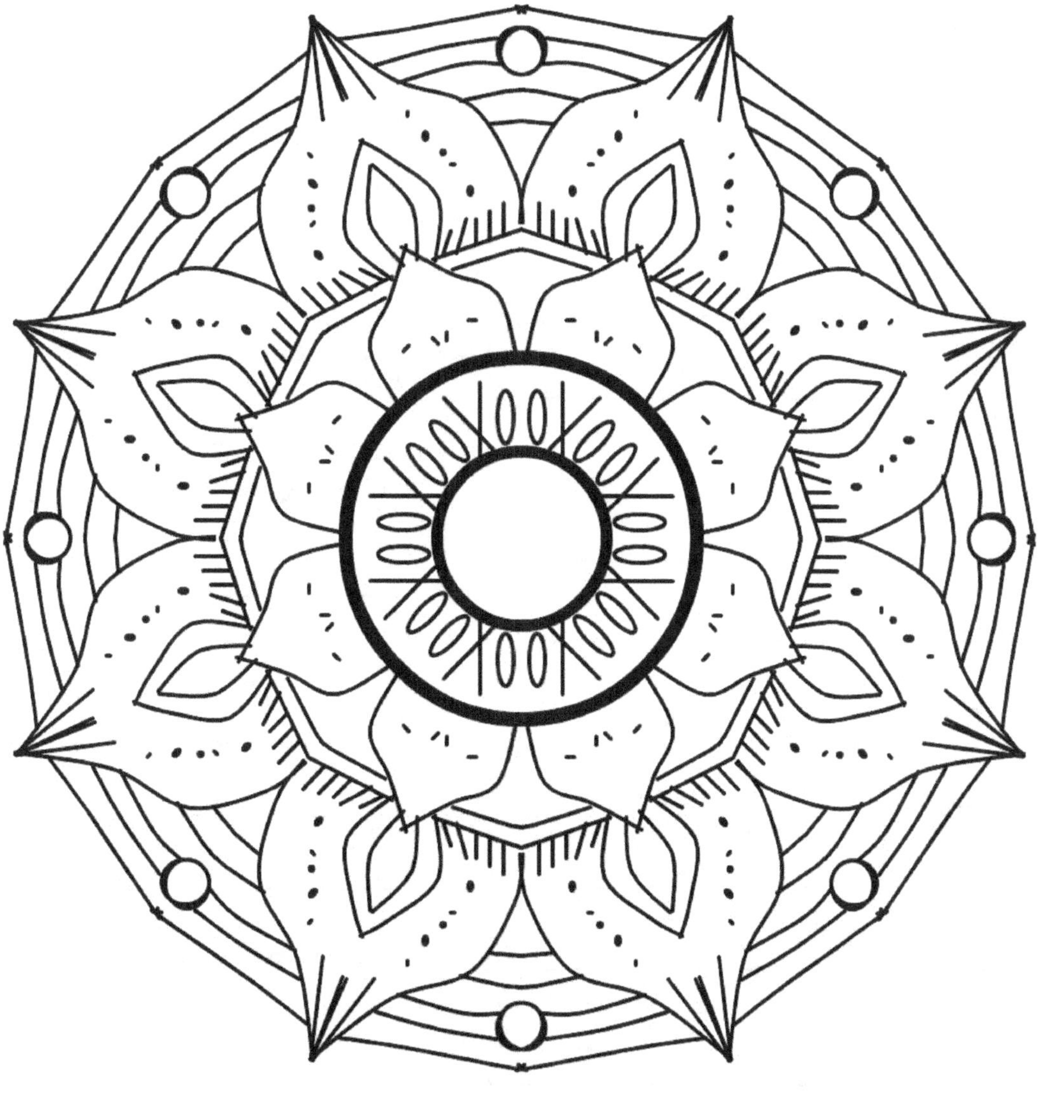

Day Thirty-one _______

5:00 ___________________________

6:00 ___________________________

7:00 ___________________________

8:00 ___________________________

9:00 ___________________________

10:00 _________________________

11:00 _________________________

Noon __________________________

1:00 ___________________________

2:00 ___________________________

3:00 ___________________________

4:00 ___________________________

5:00 ___________________________

6:00 ___________________________

7:00 ___________________________

8:00 ___________________________

9:00 ___________________________

10:00 _________________________

11:00 _________________________

Midnight ____________________

Is being forceful a bad thing?

The Workout

Exercise	Set 1	Set 2	Set 3	Set 4	Set 5	notes

Time started: _______________   Time ended: _______________

Location: ____

Feelings before training: 

Feelings after training

NUTRITION

Meal 1
time eaten: _________

Meal 2
time eaten: _________

Meal 3
time eaten: _________

Meal 4
time eaten: _________

Meal 5
time eaten: _________

Hydration

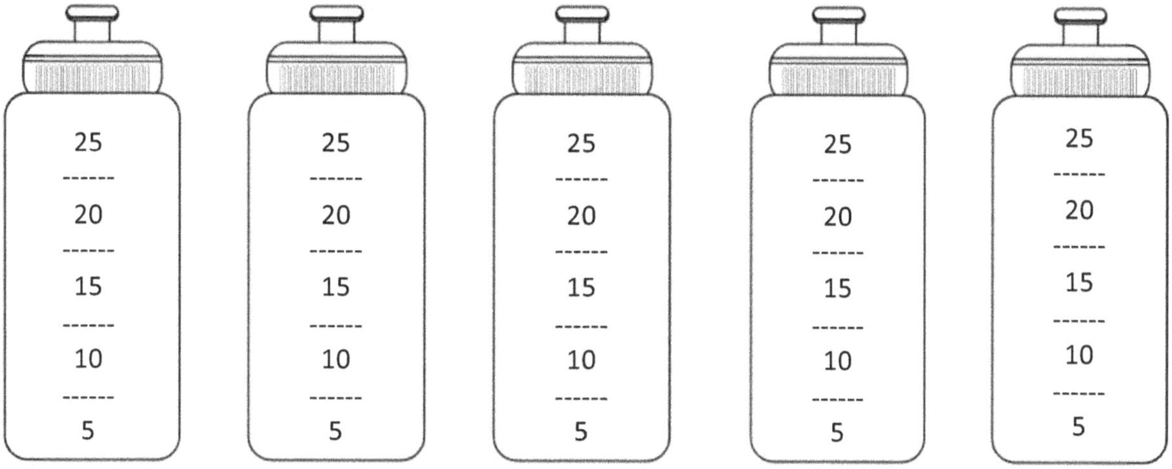

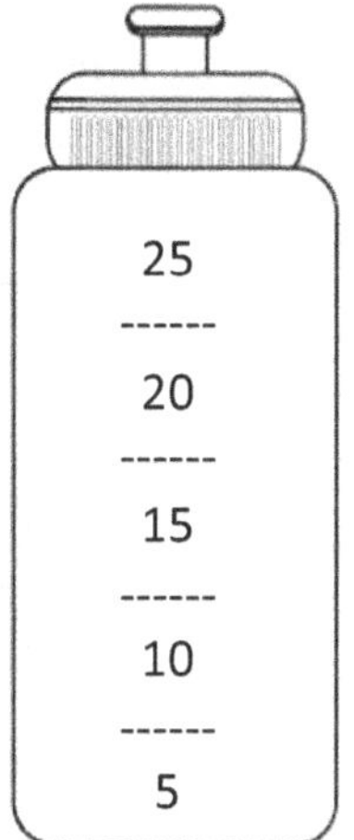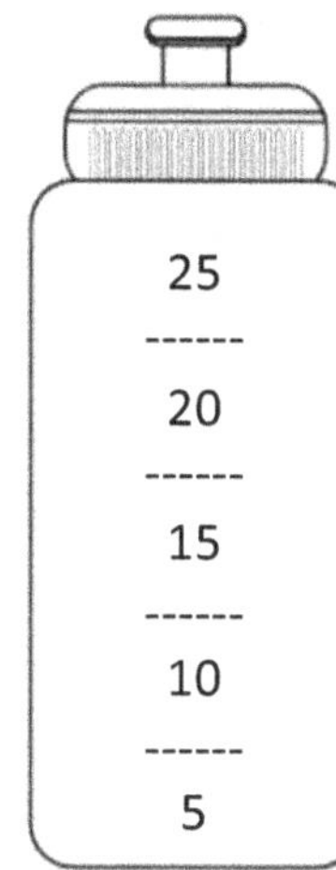

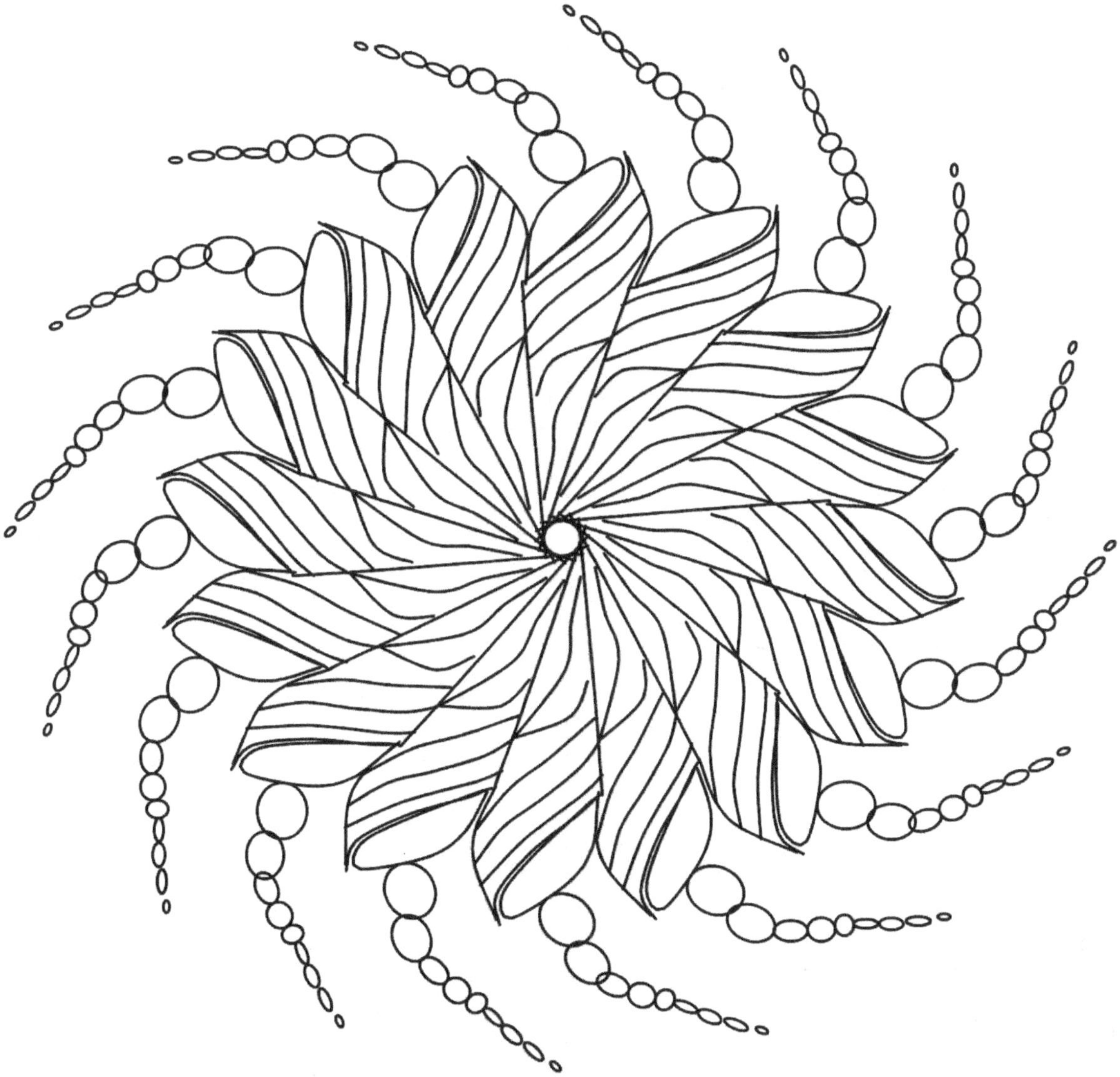

Day Thirty-two _______

5:00 _______________________

6:00 _______________________

7:00 _______________________

8:00 _______________________

9:00 _______________________

10:00 ______________________

11:00 ______________________

Noon _______________________

1:00 _______________________

2:00 _______________________

3:00 _______________________

4:00 _______________________

5:00 _______________________

6:00 _______________________

7:00 _______________________

8:00 _______________________

9:00 _______________________

10:00 ______________________

11:00 ______________________

Midnight ___________________

top priorities for today

____

____

____

____

Today's victories

What does it mean to be fervent?

____

____

____

____

____

The Stella Society Workout

Exercise	Set 1	Set 2	Set 3	Set 4	Set 5	notes

Time started: ______________ Time ended: _______________

Location: ____

Feelings before training: 😊 😐 ☹️ 😜 😠 🙁 😇 😎

Feelings after training 😊 😐 ☹️ 😜 😠 🙁 😇 😎

NUTRITION

Meal 1
time eaten: _________

Meal 2
time eaten: _________

Meal 3
time eaten: _________

Meal 4
time eaten: _________

Meal 5
time eaten: _________

Hydration

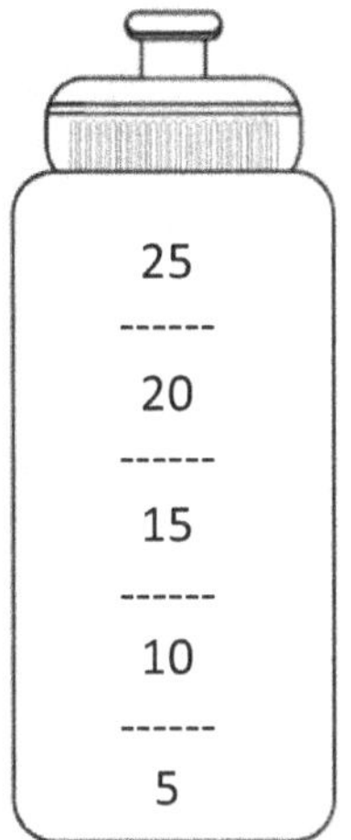
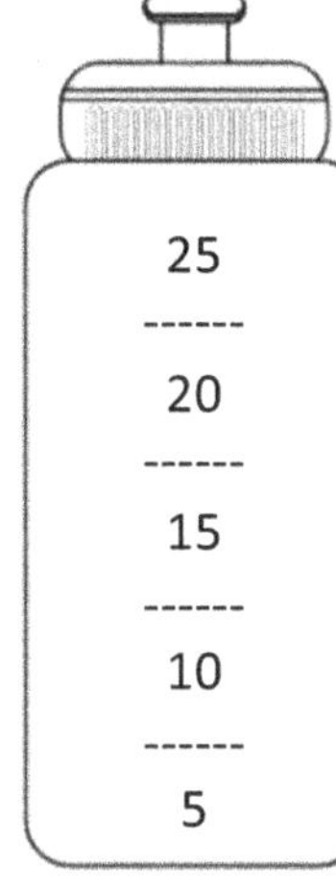
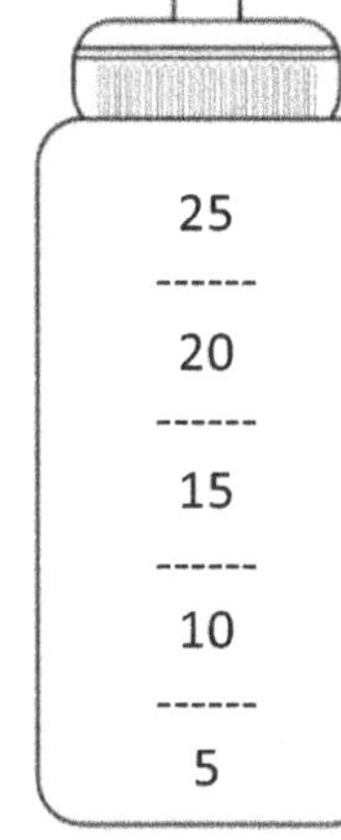
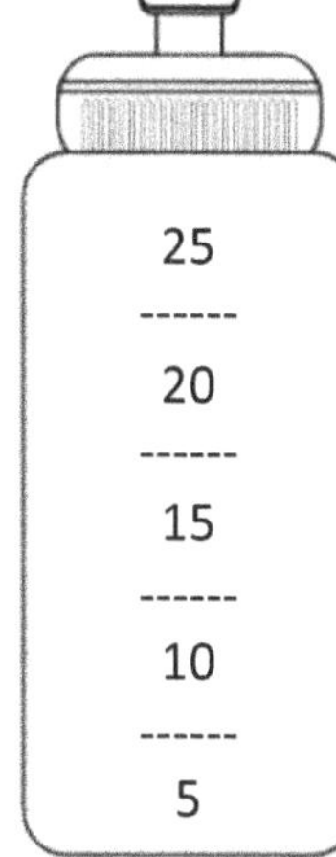
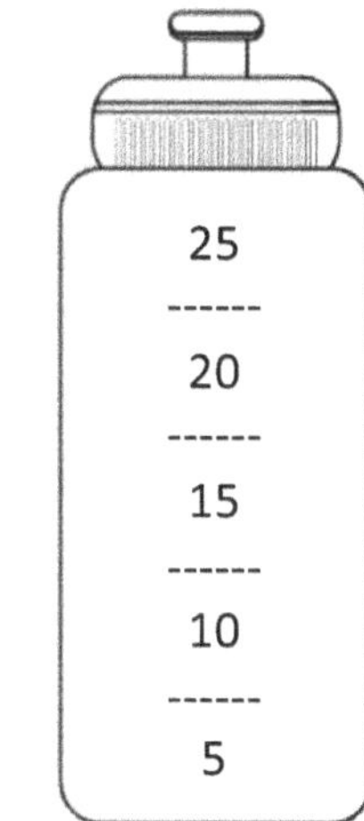

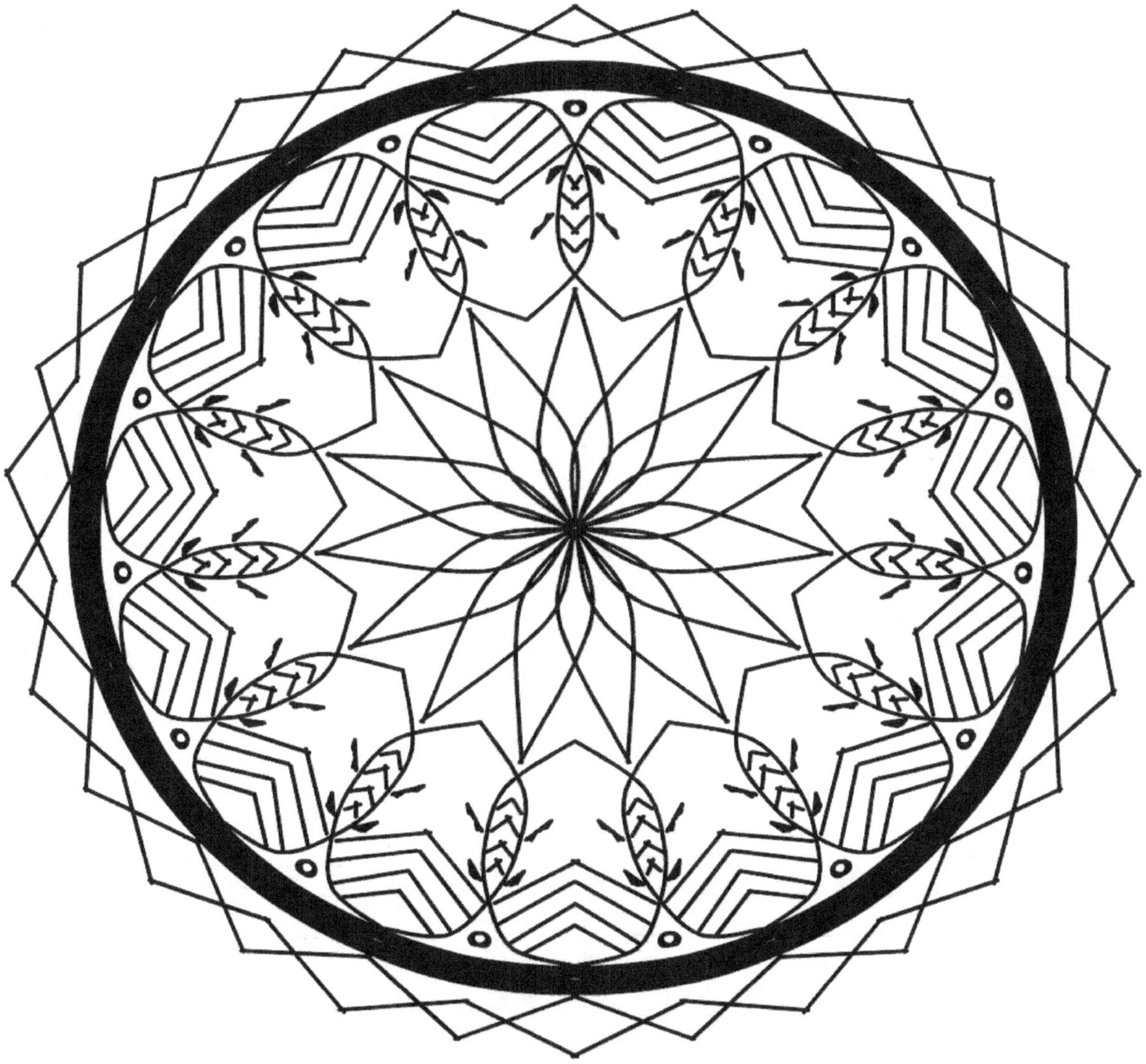

Day Thirty-three _______

5:00 __________________	top priorities for today 🎯
6:00 __________________	
7:00 __________________	__________________
8:00 __________________	__________________
9:00 __________________	__________________
10:00 _________________	__________________
11:00 _________________	__________________
Noon __________________	
1:00 __________________	Today's victories 🏆
2:00 __________________	
3:00 __________________	
4:00 __________________	
5:00 __________________	
6:00 __________________	How are you glowing today?
7:00 __________________	
8:00 __________________	__________________
9:00 __________________	__________________
10:00 _________________	__________________
11:00 _________________	__________________
Midnight _______________	__________________

The Workout

Exercise	Set 1	Set 2	Set 3	Set 4	Set 5	notes

Time started: _______________ Time ended: _______________

Location: ____

Feelings before training: 🙂 😐 🙁 😜 😠 😕 😊 😎

Feelings after training 🙂 😐 🙁 😜 😠 😕 😊 😎

NUTRITION

Meal 1

time eaten: _________

Meal 2

time eaten: _________

Meal 3

time eaten: _________

Meal 4

time eaten: _________

Meal 5

time eaten: _________

Hydration

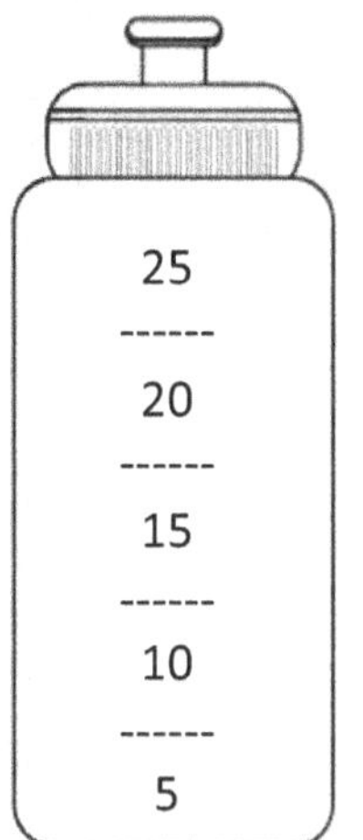
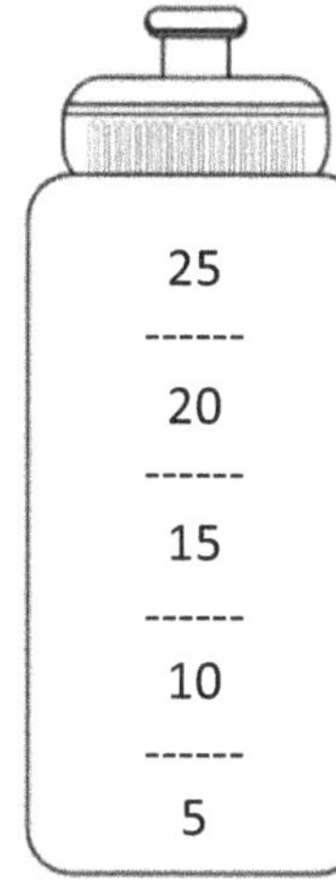
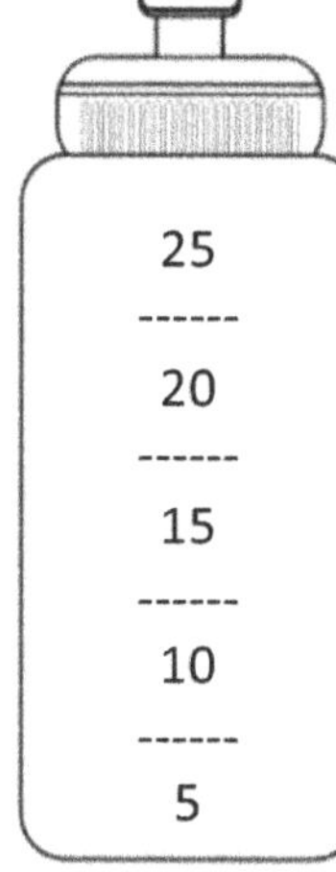
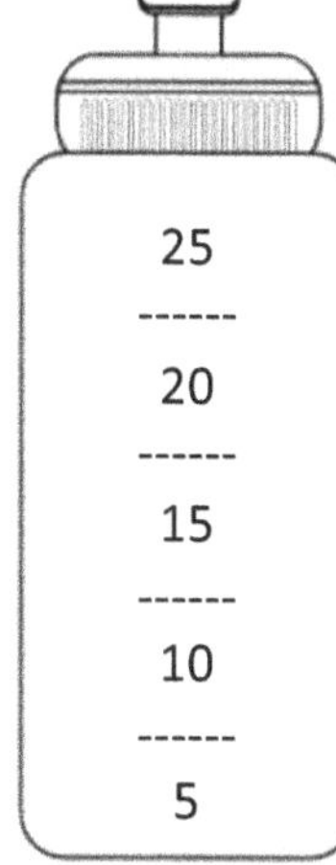
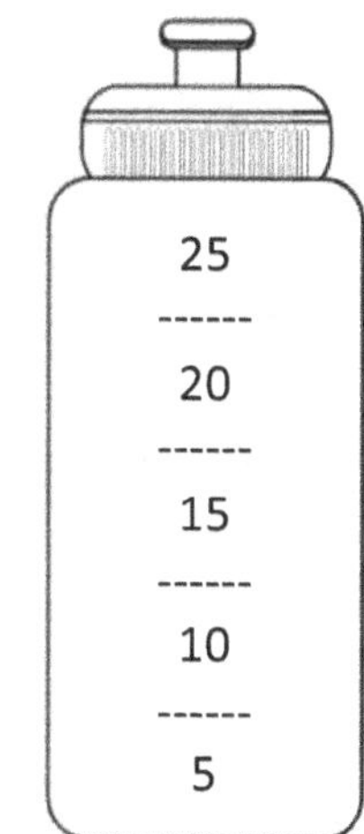

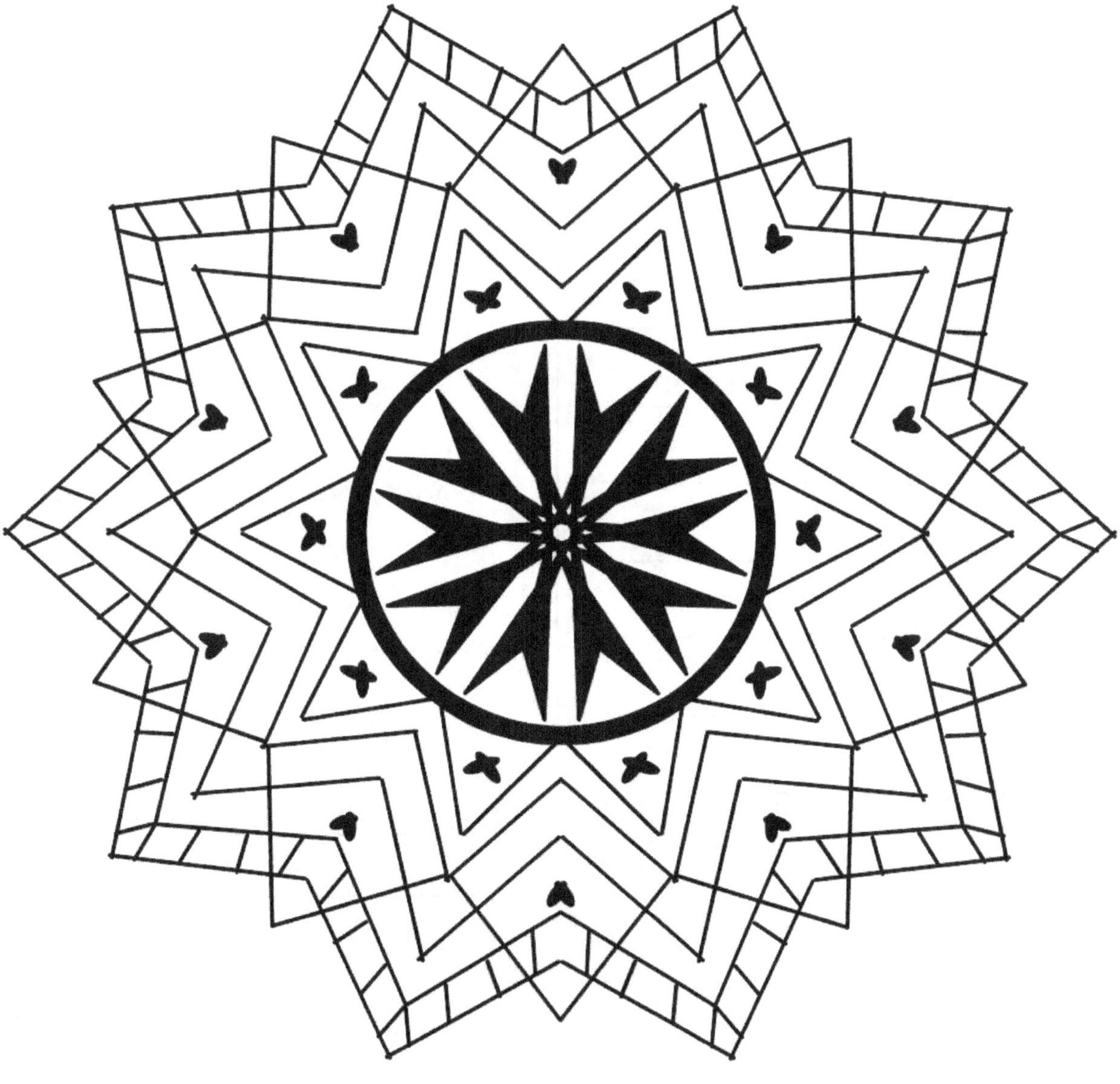

Day Thirty-four _______

5:00 _______________________

6:00 _______________________

7:00 _______________________

8:00 _______________________

9:00 _______________________

10:00 ______________________

11:00 ______________________

Noon _______________________

1:00 _______________________

2:00 _______________________

3:00 _______________________

4:00 _______________________

5:00 _______________________

6:00 _______________________

7:00 _______________________

8:00 _______________________

9:00 _______________________

10:00 ______________________

11:00 ______________________

Midnight ___________________

Today's victories

What are you dedicated to
do at this moment?

The Stella Society Workout

Exercise	Set 1	Set 2	Set 3	Set 4	Set 5	notes

Time started: _____________   Time ended: _______________

Location: ____

Feelings before training:

Feelings after training

NUTRITION

Meal 1

time eaten: _________

Meal 2

time eaten: _________

Meal 3

time eaten: _________

Meal 4

time eaten: _________

Meal 5

time eaten: _________

Hydration

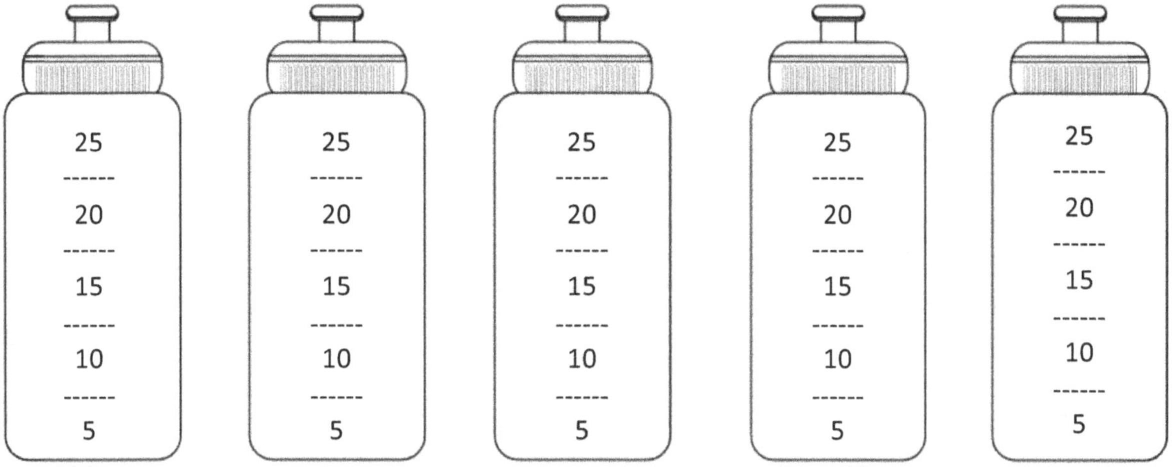

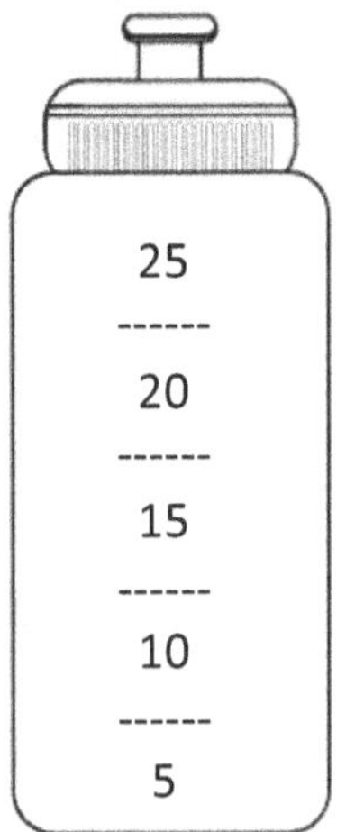 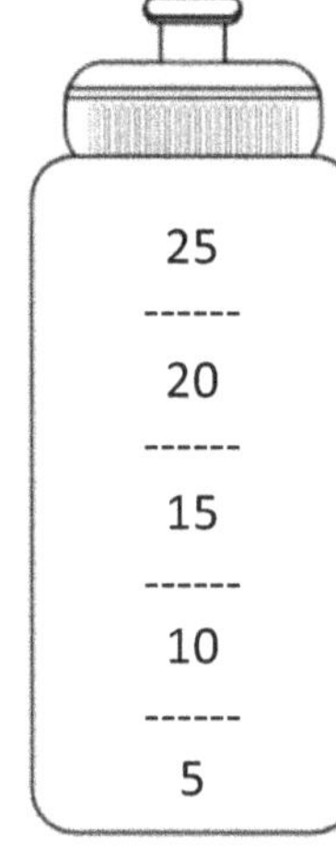 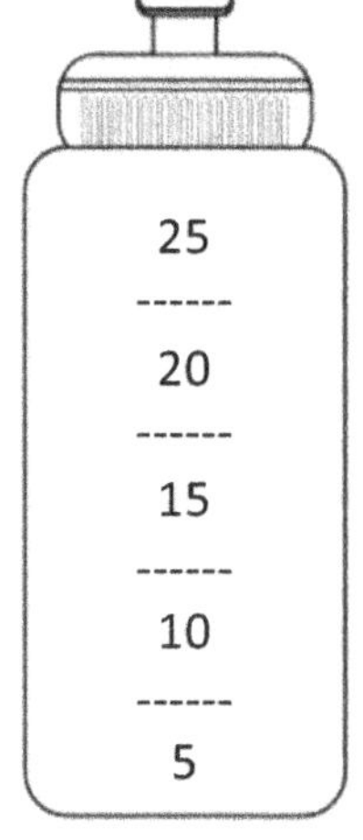

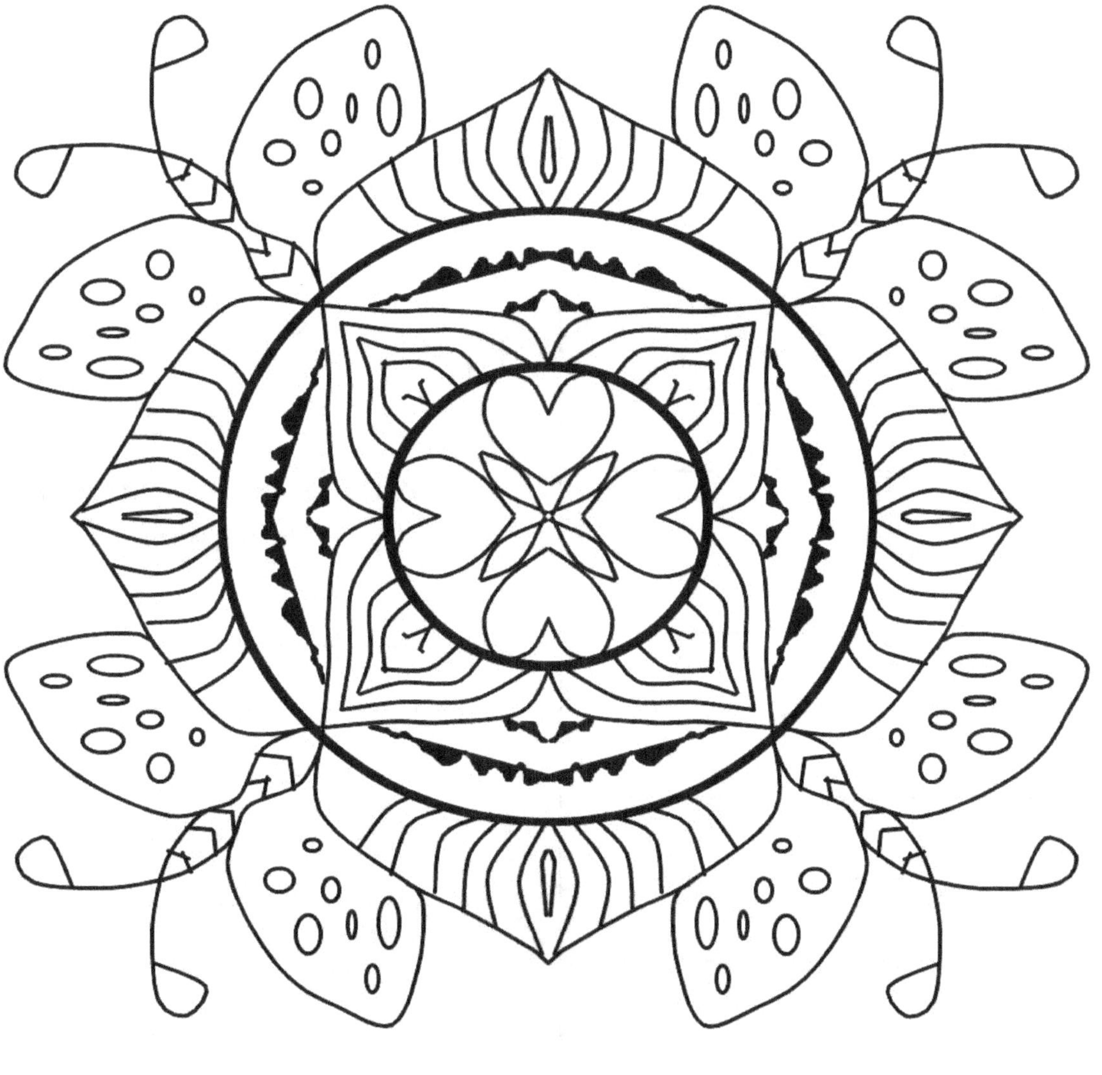

Day Thirty-five _______

5:00 _______________________

6:00 _______________________

7:00 _______________________

8:00 _______________________

9:00 _______________________

10:00 ______________________

11:00 ______________________

Noon _______________________

1:00 _______________________

2:00 _______________________

3:00 _______________________

4:00 _______________________

5:00 _______________________

6:00 _______________________

7:00 _______________________

8:00 _______________________

9:00 _______________________

10:00 ______________________

11:00 ______________________

Midnight __________________

____

____

____

____

Today's victories

Who is more determined than you?

____

____

____

____

____

____

The Stella Society Workout

Exercise	Set 1	Set 2	Set 3	Set 4	Set 5	notes

Time started: _____________ Time ended: _______________

Location: ____

Feelings before training:

Feelings after training

NUTRITION

Meal 1

time eaten: _________

Meal 2

time eaten: _________

Meal 3

time eaten: _________

Meal 4

time eaten: _________

Meal 5

time eaten: _________

Hydration

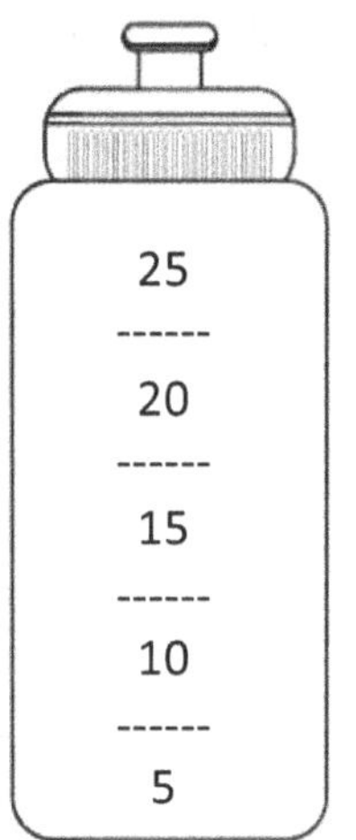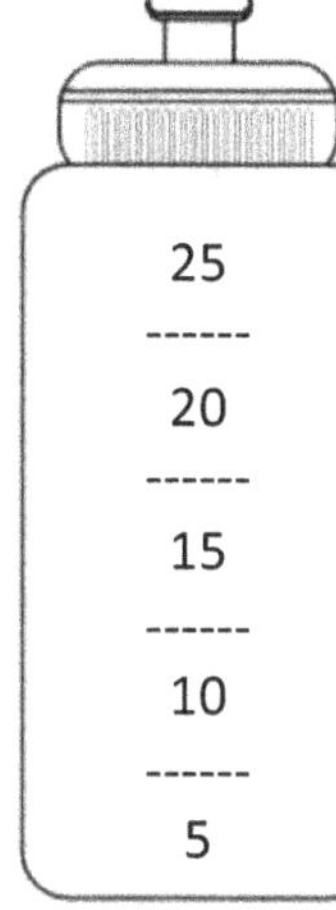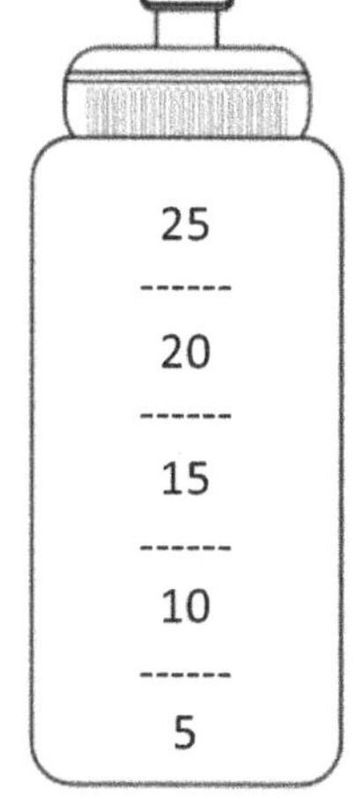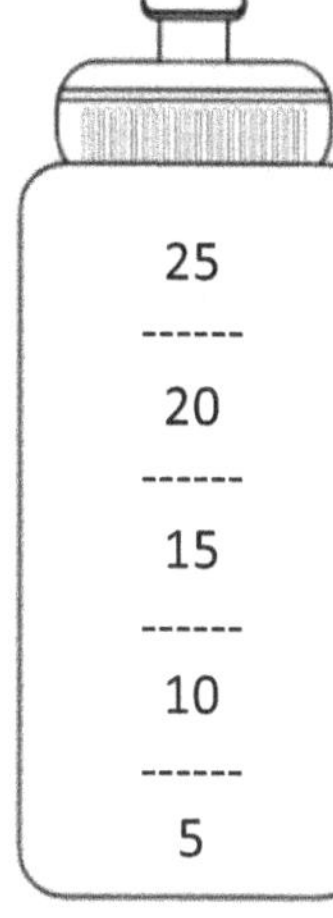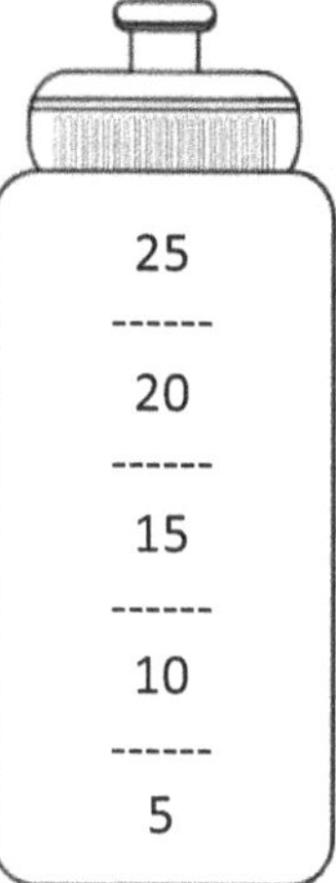

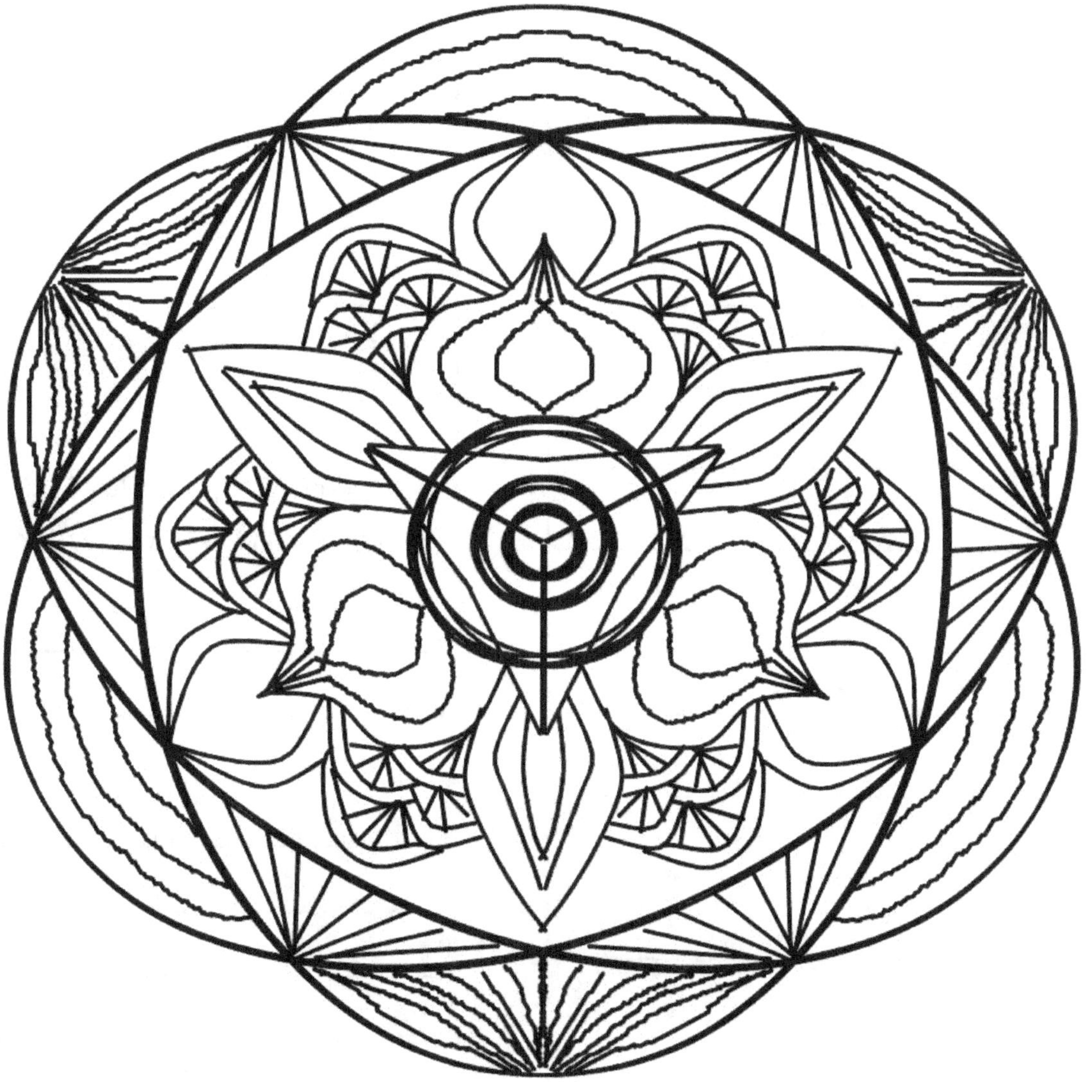

Day Thirty-six ______

5:00 ______________________

6:00 ______________________

7:00 ______________________

8:00 ______________________

9:00 ______________________

10:00 ______________________

11:00 ______________________

Noon ______________________

1:00 ______________________

2:00 ______________________

3:00 ______________________

4:00 ______________________

5:00 ______________________

6:00 ______________________

7:00 ______________________

8:00 ______________________

9:00 ______________________

10:00 ______________________

11:00 ______________________

Midnight __________________

top priorities for today

Today's victories

Who needs your acceptance
of change and why?

The Stella Society Workout

Exercise	Set 1	Set 2	Set 3	Set 4	Set 5	notes

Time started: _______________   Time ended: _______________

Location: ____

Feelings before training: 😊 😐 ☹️ 😜 😠 😕 😊 😎

Feelings after training 😊 😐 ☹️ 😜 😠 😕 😊 😎

NUTRITION

Meal 1

time eaten: _________

Meal 2

time eaten: _________

Meal 3

time eaten: _________

Meal 4

time eaten: _________

Meal 5

time eaten: _________

Hydration

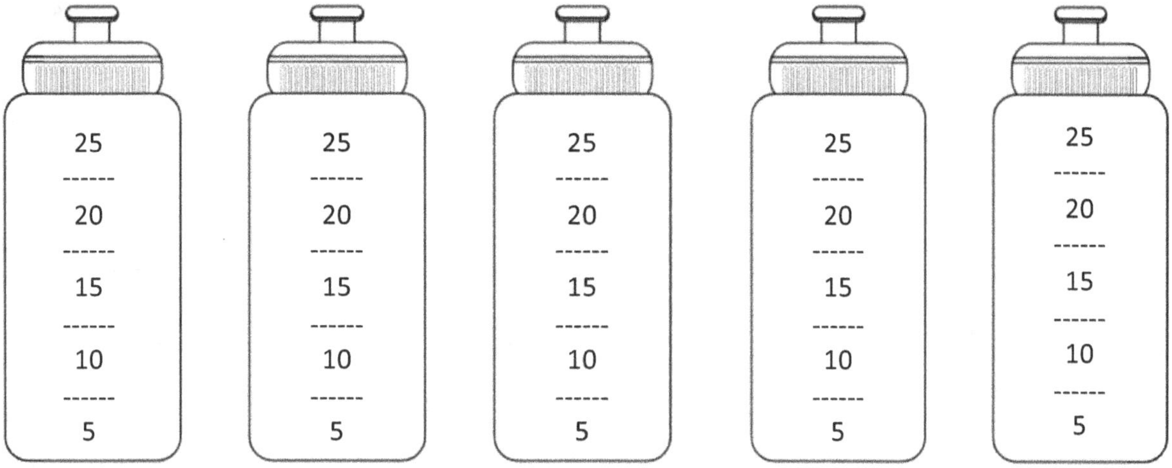

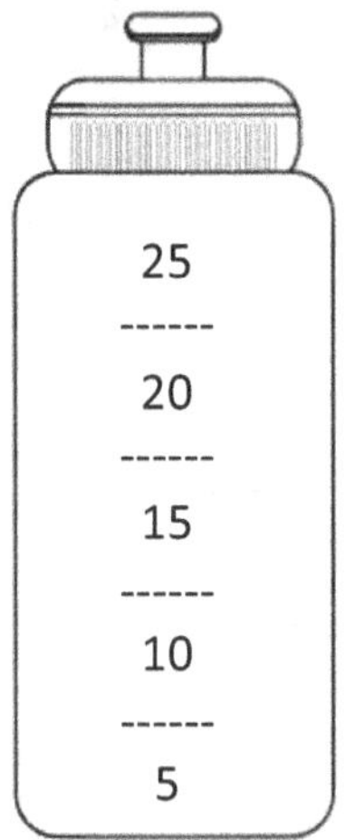 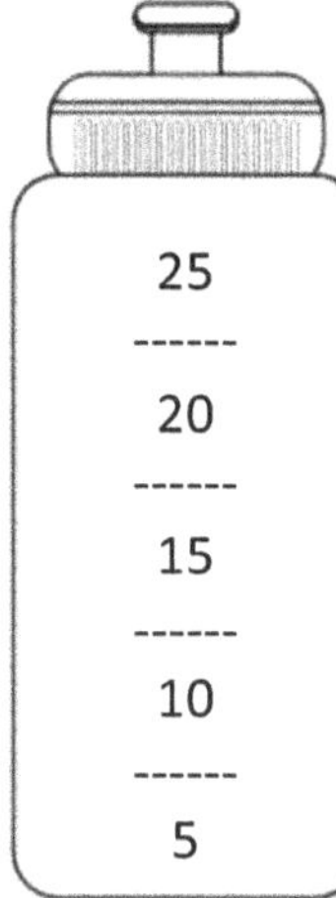 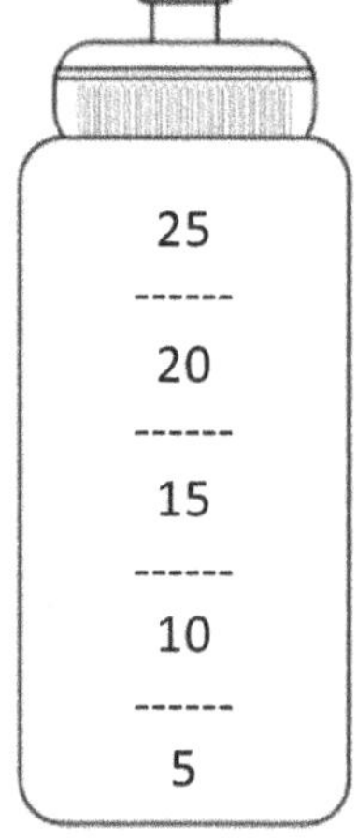 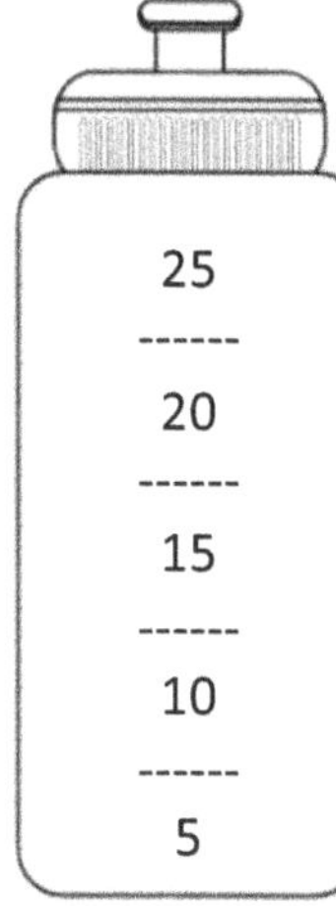 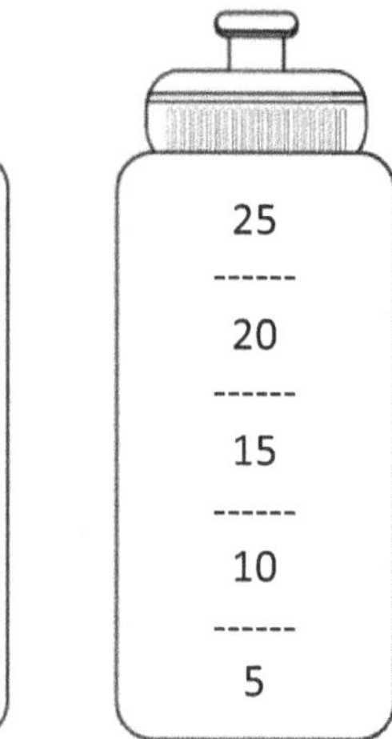

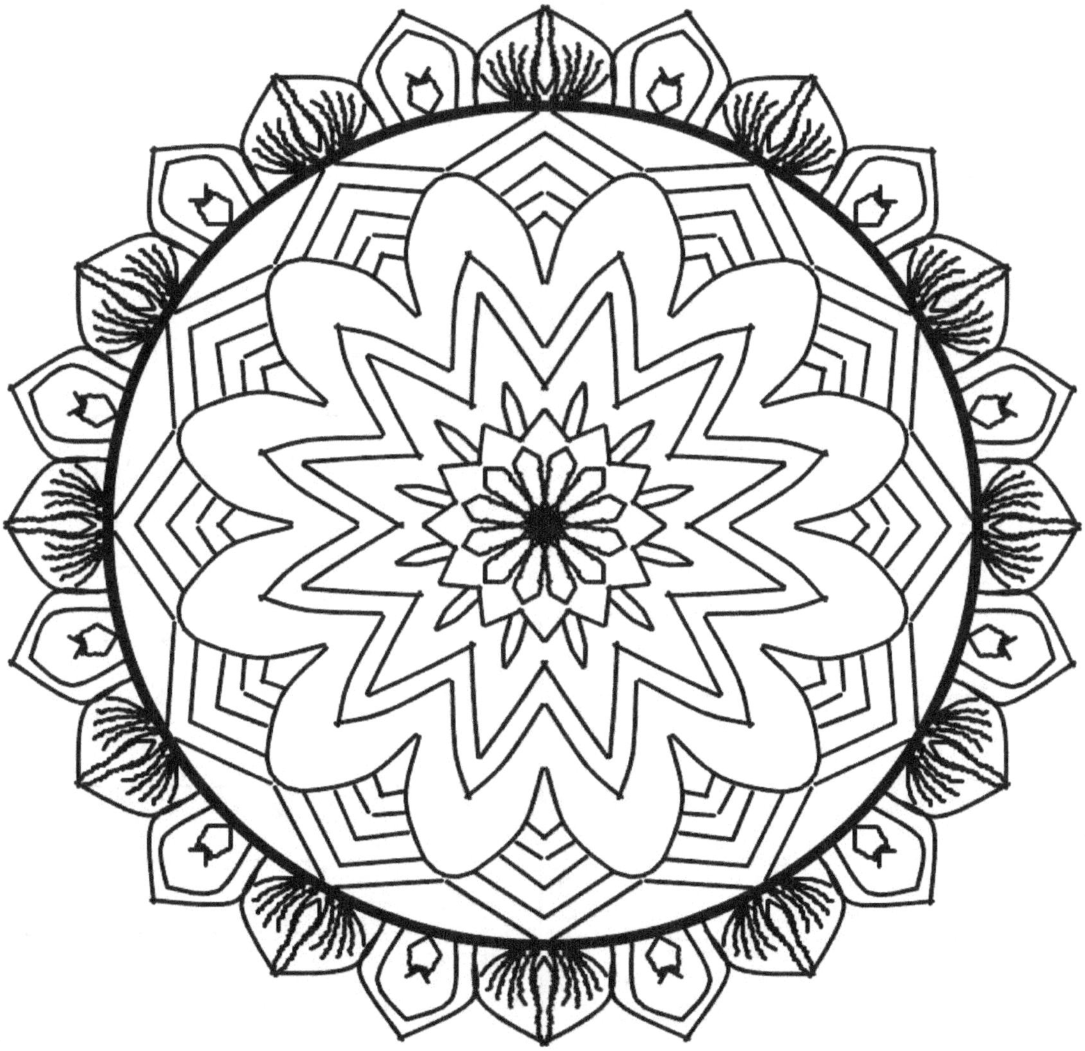

Day Thirty-seven _______

5:00 _______________________

6:00 _______________________

7:00 _______________________

8:00 _______________________

9:00 _______________________

10:00 ______________________

11:00 ______________________

Noon _______________________

1:00 _______________________

2:00 _______________________

3:00 _______________________

4:00 _______________________

5:00 _______________________

6:00 _______________________

7:00 _______________________

8:00 _______________________

9:00 _______________________

10:00 ______________________

11:00 ______________________

Midnight ___________________

____

____

____

____

Today's victories

How will you be captivating?

The Stella Society Workout

Exercise	Set 1	Set 2	Set 3	Set 4	Set 5	notes

Time started: _____________   Time ended: _____________

Location: ____

Feelings before training: 🙂 😐 🙁 😜 😠 😕 😊 😎

Feelings after training 🙂 😐 🙁 😜 😠 😕 😊 😎

NUTRITION

Meal 1
time eaten: _________

Meal 2
time eaten: _________

Meal 3
time eaten: _________

Meal 4
time eaten: _________

Meal 5
time eaten: _________

Hydration

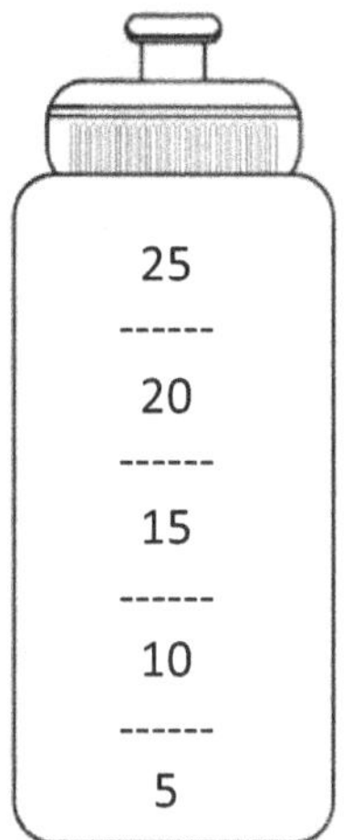
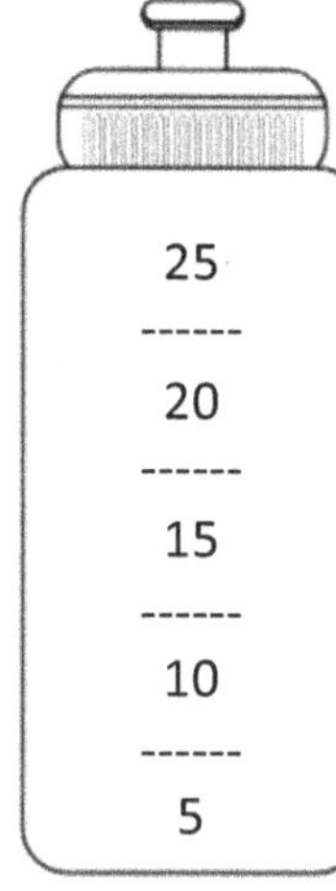
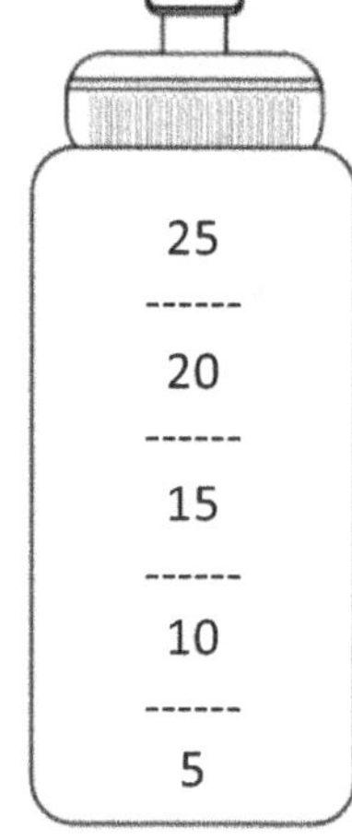
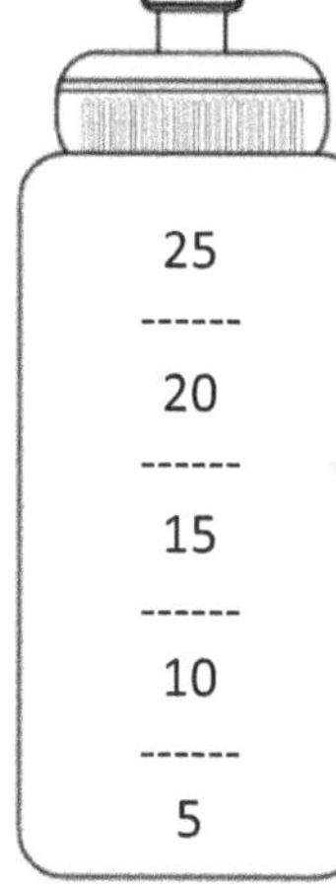
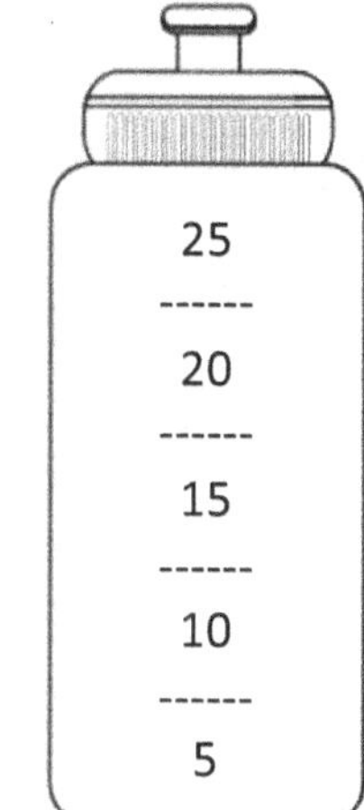

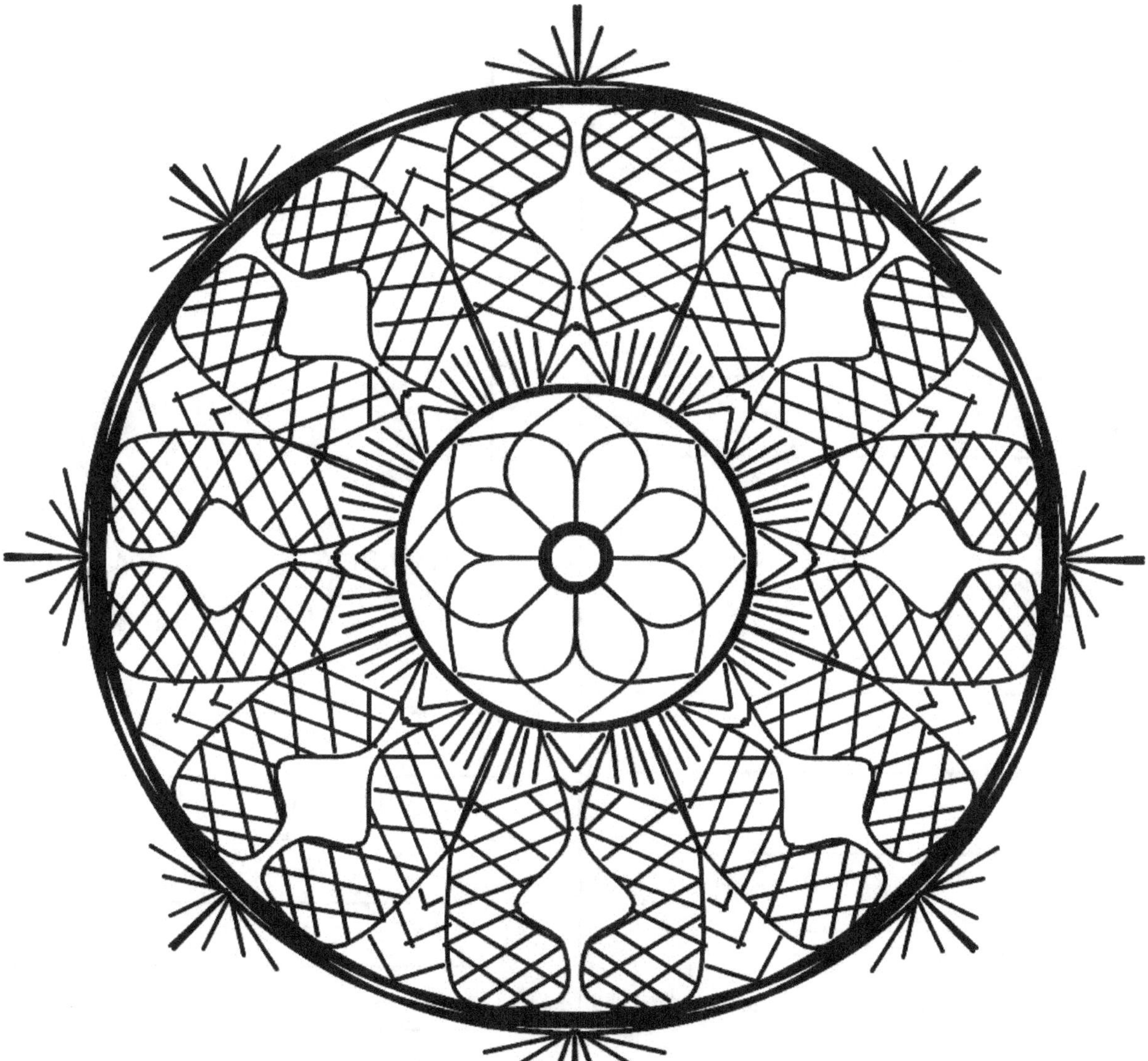

Day Thirty-eight _______

5:00 _______________________

6:00 _______________________

7:00 _______________________

8:00 _______________________

9:00 _______________________

10:00 _______________________

11:00 _______________________

Noon _______________________

1:00 _______________________

2:00 _______________________

3:00 _______________________

4:00 _______________________

5:00 _______________________

6:00 _______________________

7:00 _______________________

8:00 _______________________

9:00 _______________________

10:00 _______________________

11:00 _______________________

Midnight _______________________

____
____
____
____
____

What does it mean to be alluring?

____
____
____
____
____
____
____

The Stella Society Workout

Exercise	Set 1	Set 2	Set 3	Set 4	Set 5	notes

Time started: ____________   Time ended: ____________

Location: ____

Feelings before training:

Feelings after training

NUTRITION

Meal 1

time eaten: _________

Meal 2

time eaten: _________

Meal 3

time eaten: _________

Meal 4

time eaten: _________

Meal 5

time eaten: _________

Hydration

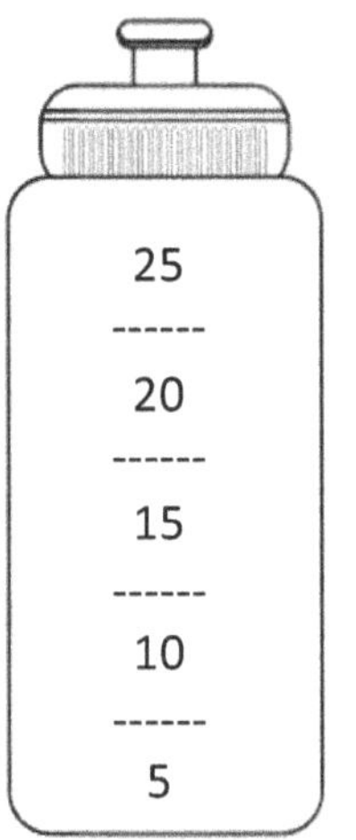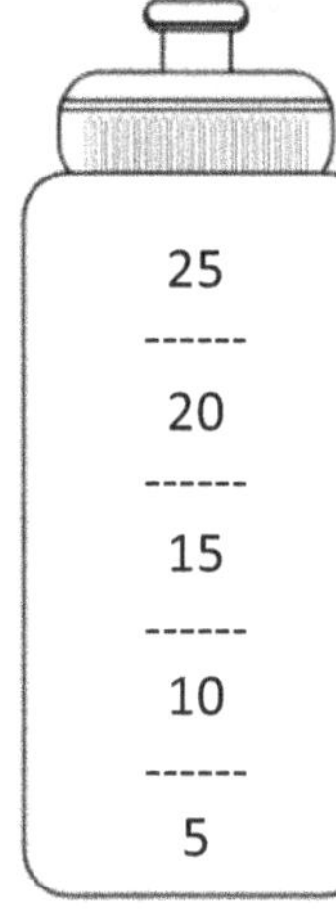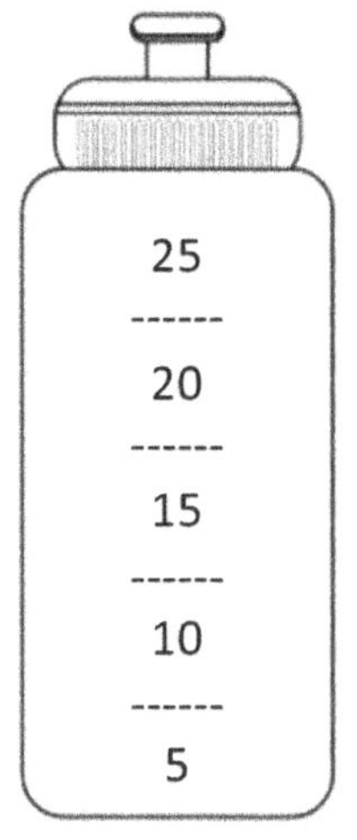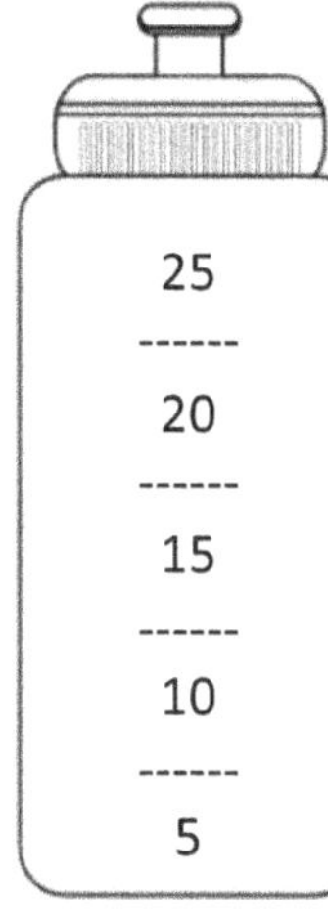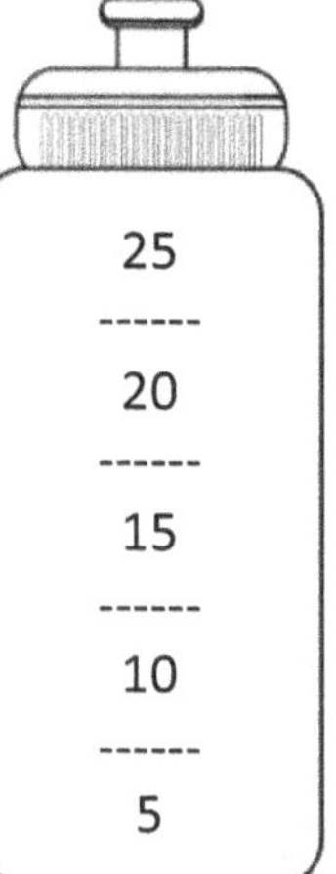

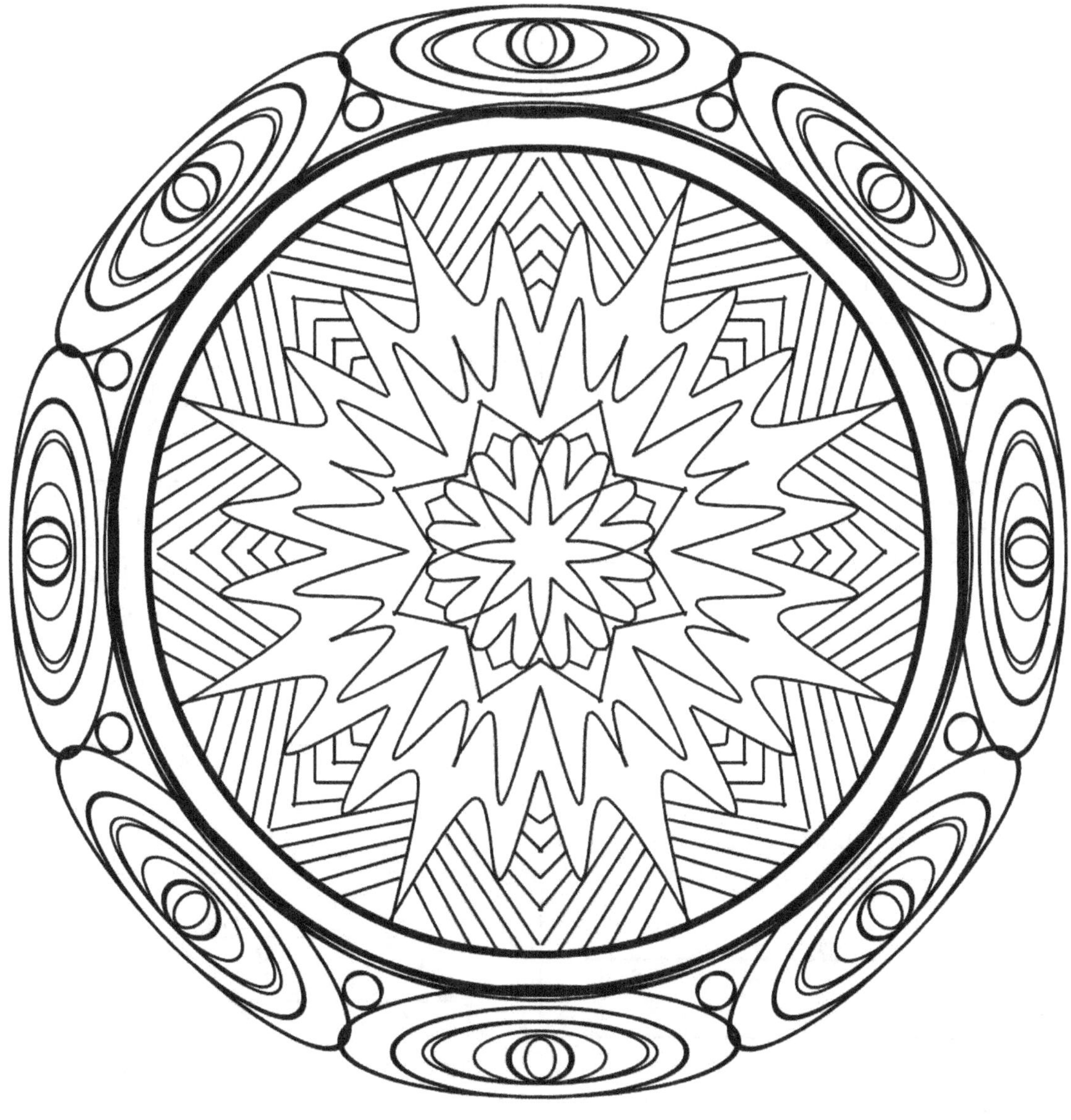

Day Thirty-nine _______

5:00 _______________________

6:00 _______________________

7:00 _______________________

8:00 _______________________

9:00 _______________________

10:00 _______________________

11:00 _______________________

Noon _______________________

1:00 _______________________

2:00 _______________________

3:00 _______________________

4:00 _______________________

5:00 _______________________

6:00 _______________________

7:00 _______________________

8:00 _______________________

9:00 _______________________

10:00 _______________________

11:00 _______________________

Midnight ___________________

top priorities for today

____

____

____

____

Today's victories

How will you be the best
version of you?

____

____

____

____

____

____

The *Stella Society* Workout

Exercise	Set 1	Set 2	Set 3	Set 4	Set 5	notes

Time started: _______________   Time ended: _______________

Location: ____

Feelings before training: 😊 😐 ☹ 😜 😠 😒 😊 😎

Feelings after training 😊 😐 ☹ 😜 😠 😒 😊 😎

NUTRITION

Meal 1
time eaten: _________

Meal 2
time eaten: _________

Meal 3
time eaten: _________

Meal 4
time eaten: _________

Meal 5
time eaten: _________

Hydration

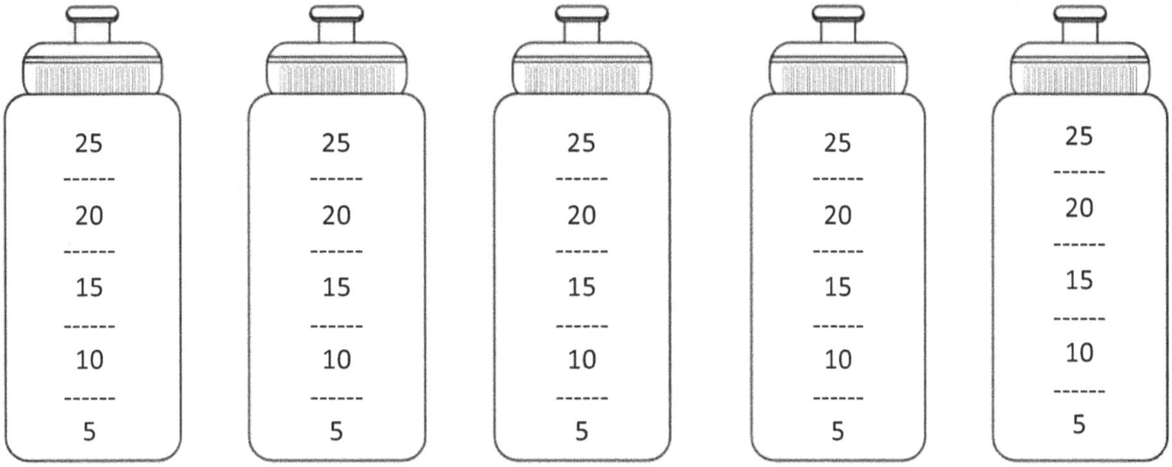

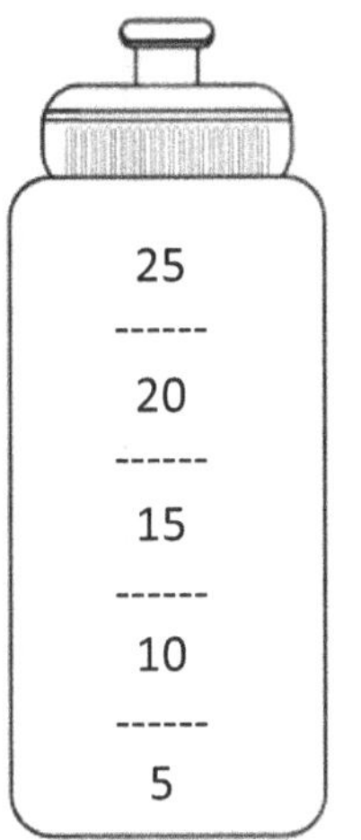
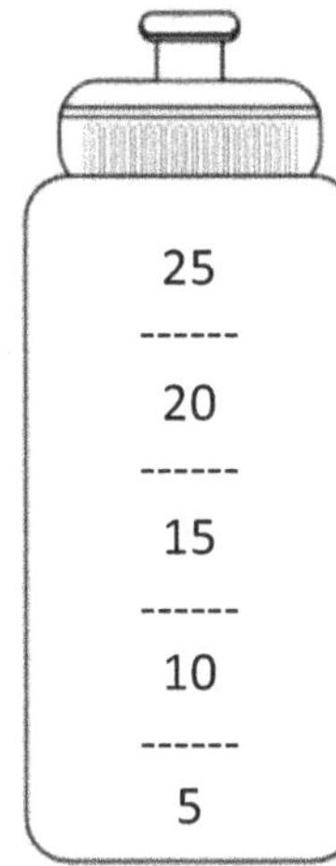
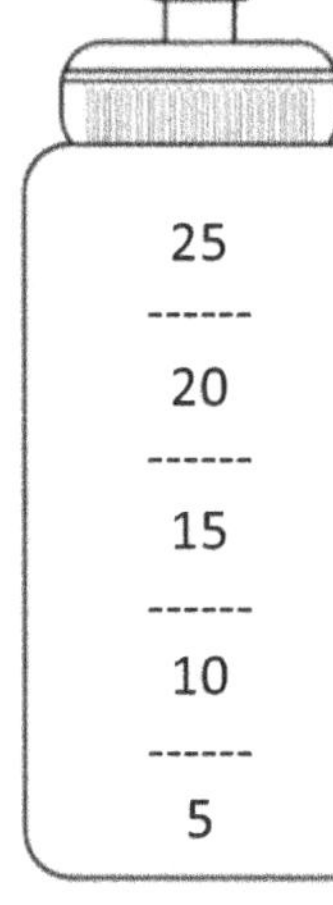

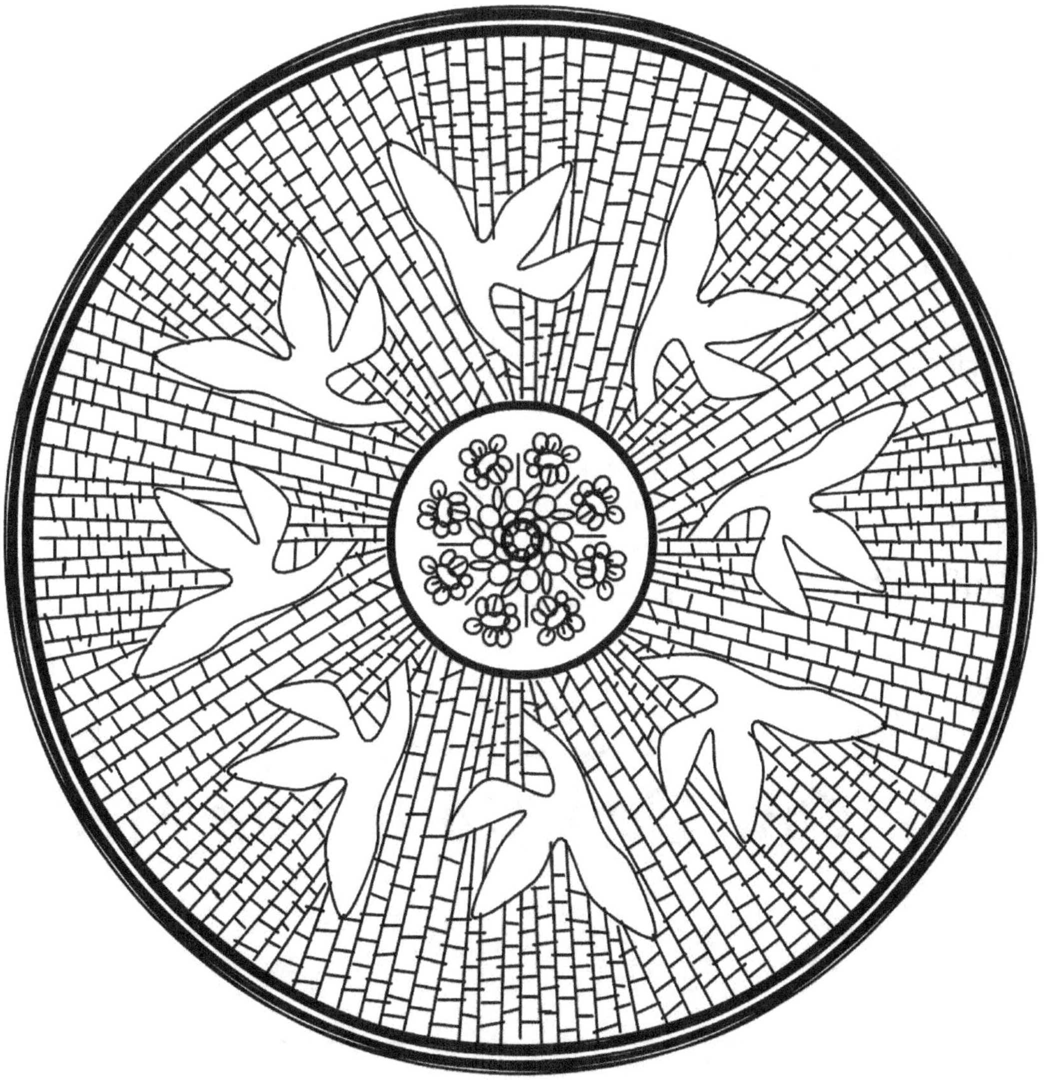

Measurements

DATE: __________

Weight: ______

Neck ______

Shoulders ______

Chest ______

Bicep / upper arm left _______ right _______

Forearm left _______ right ______

Waist ______

Hips ______

Thighs left _______ right ______

Calf left _______ right ______

**Only I Can Change My Life,
No One Can Do It For Me!**

Day Forty ______

5:00 ____________	

5:00 ____________________

6:00 ____________________

7:00 ____________________

8:00 ____________________

9:00 ____________________

10:00 ____________________

11:00 ____________________

Noon ____________________

1:00 ____________________

2:00 ____________________

3:00 ____________________

4:00 ____________________

5:00 ____________________

6:00 ____________________

7:00 ____________________

8:00 ____________________

9:00 ____________________

10:00 ____________________

11:00 ____________________

Midnight ____________________

top priorities for today

Today's victories

Do you believe in magic or miracles?

The Stella Society Workout

Exercise	Set 1	Set 2	Set 3	Set 4	Set 5	notes

Time started: _____________ Time ended: _______________

Location: ____

Feelings before training: 😊 😐 ☹ 😜 😠 😕 😇 😎

Feelings after training 😊 😐 ☹ 😜 😠 😕 😇 😎

NUTRITION

Meal 1

time eaten: _________

Meal 2

time eaten: _________

Meal 3

time eaten: _________

Meal 4

time eaten: _________

Meal 5

time eaten: _________

Hydration

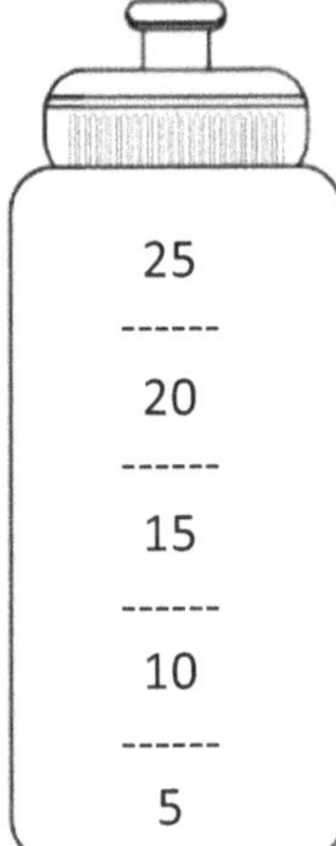
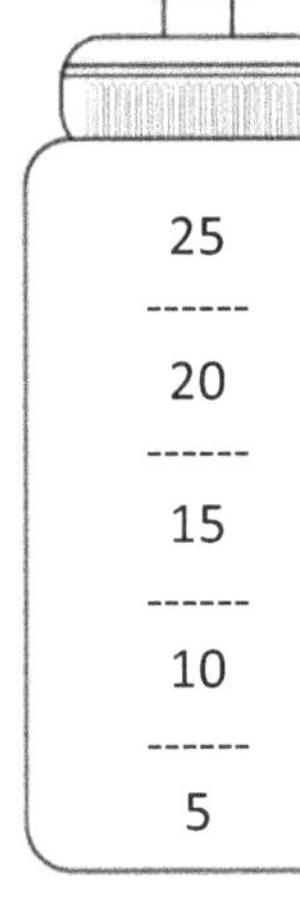
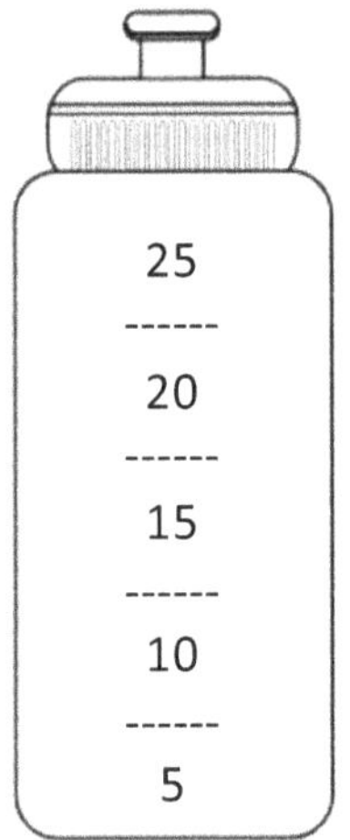
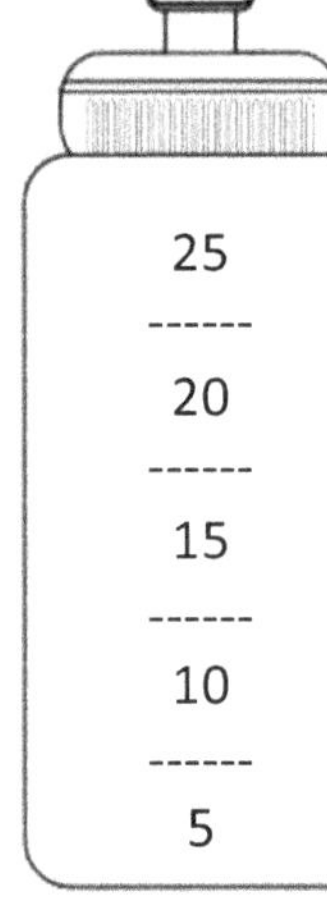
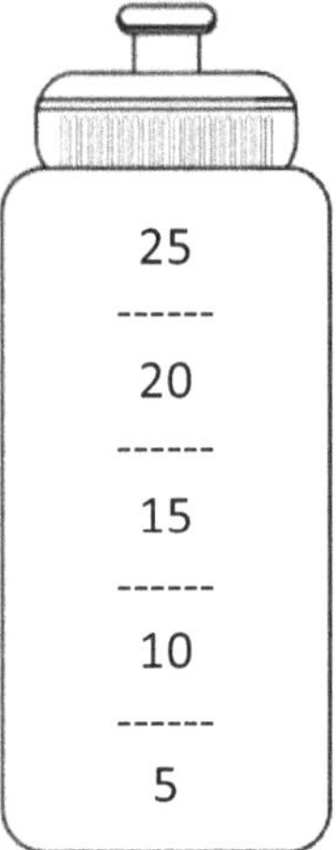

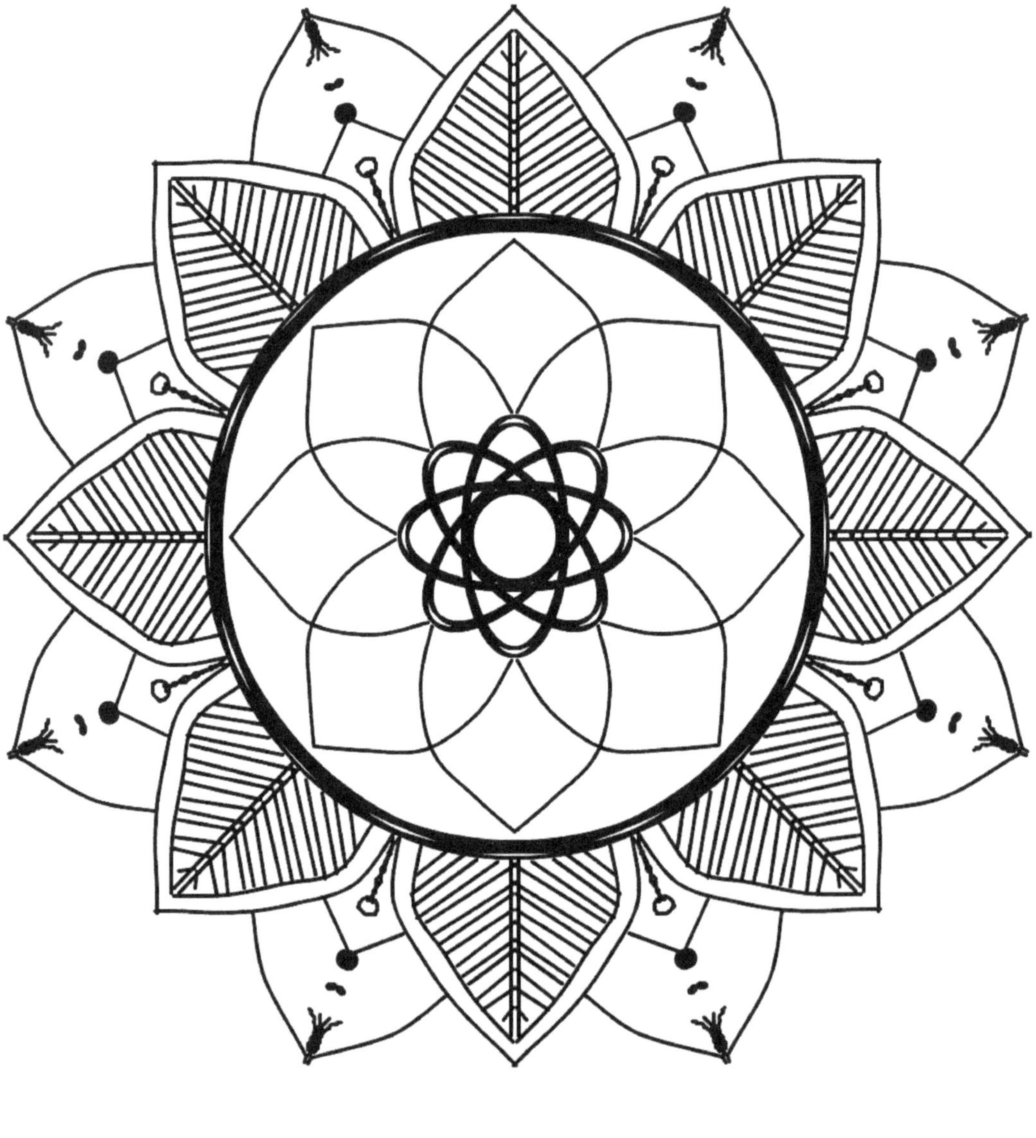

Day Forty-one ______

5:00 _____________________

6:00 _____________________

7:00 _____________________

8:00 _____________________

9:00 _____________________

10:00 _____________________

11:00 _____________________

Noon _____________________

1:00 _____________________

2:00 _____________________

3:00 _____________________

4:00 _____________________

5:00 _____________________

6:00 _____________________

7:00 _____________________

8:00 _____________________

9:00 _____________________

10:00 _____________________

11:00 _____________________

Midnight _____________________

top priorities for today 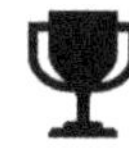

____

____

____

____

Today's victories

What is one thing you want to do forever?

____

____

____

____

____

____

The Stella Society Workout

Exercise	Set 1	Set 2	Set 3	Set 4	Set 5	notes

Time started: _____________ Time ended: ______________

Location: ____

Feelings before training:

Feelings after training

NUTRITION

Meal 1

time eaten: _________

Meal 2

time eaten: _________

Meal 3

time eaten: _________

Meal 4

time eaten: _________

Meal 5

time eaten: _________

Hydration

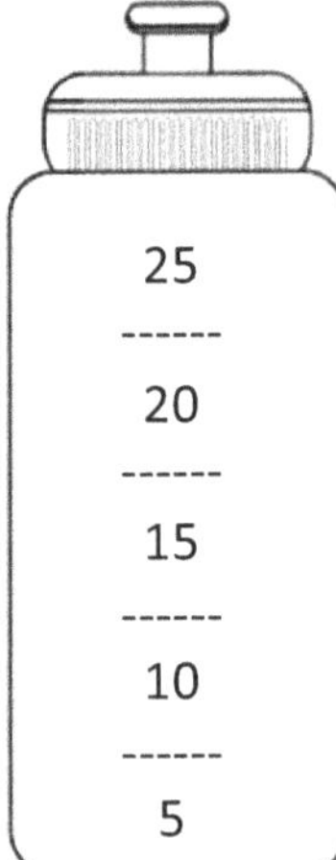

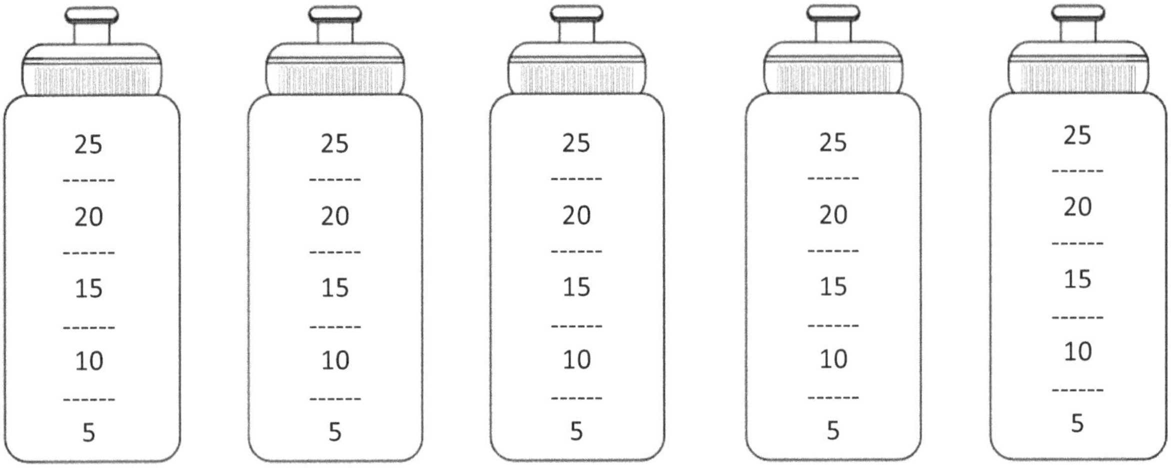

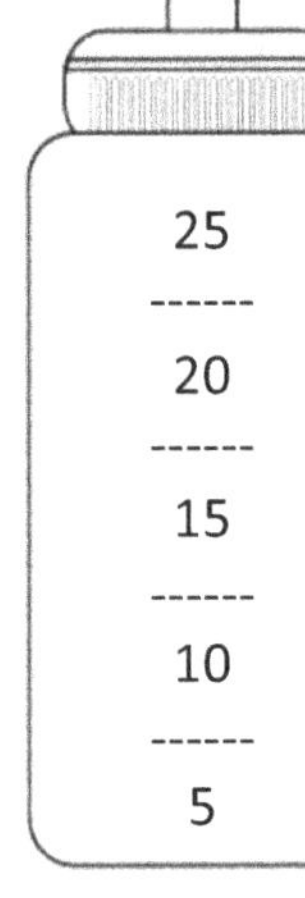

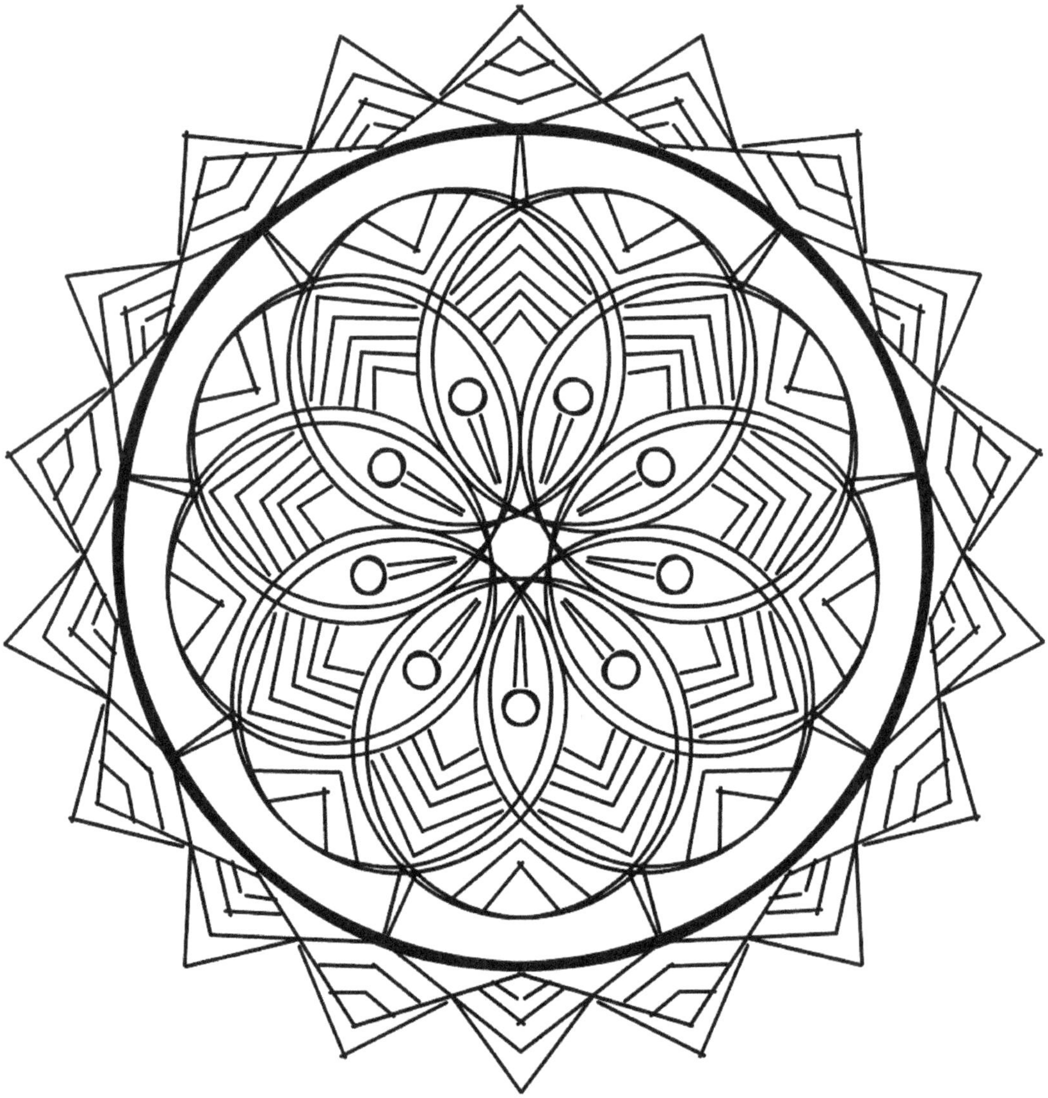

Day Forty-two _______

top priorities for today 

5:00 _____________________

6:00 _____________________

7:00 _____________________

8:00 _____________________

9:00 _____________________

10:00 ____________________

11:00 ____________________

Noon _____________________

1:00 _____________________

2:00 _____________________

3:00 _____________________

4:00 _____________________

5:00 _____________________

6:00 _____________________

7:00 _____________________

8:00 _____________________

9:00 _____________________

10:00 ____________________

11:00 ____________________

Midnight _________________

Today's victories 🏆

What was your biggest
victory in the last 40 days?

The Stella Society Workout

Exercise	Set 1	Set 2	Set 3	Set 4	Set 5	notes

Time started: _____________   Time ended: _______________

Location: ____

Feelings before training:

Feelings after training

NUTRITION

Meal 1
time eaten: _________

Meal 2
time eaten: _________

Meal 3
time eaten: _________

Meal 4
time eaten: _________

Meal 5
time eaten: _________

Hydration

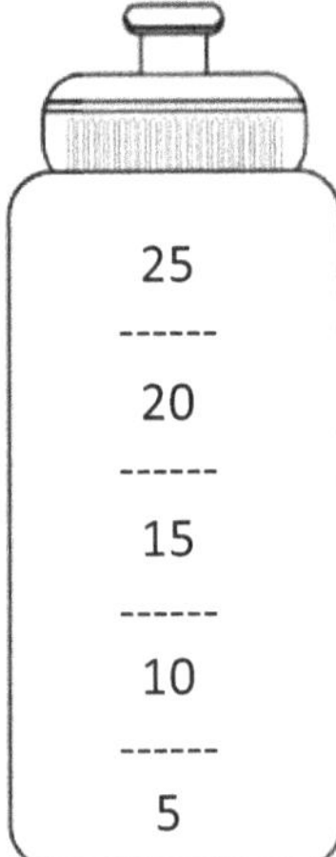

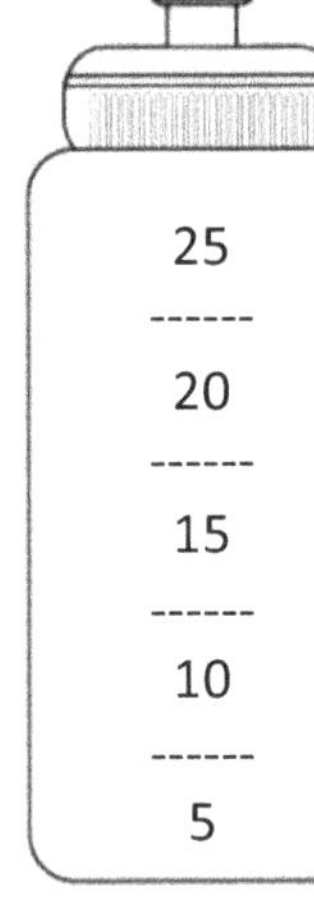

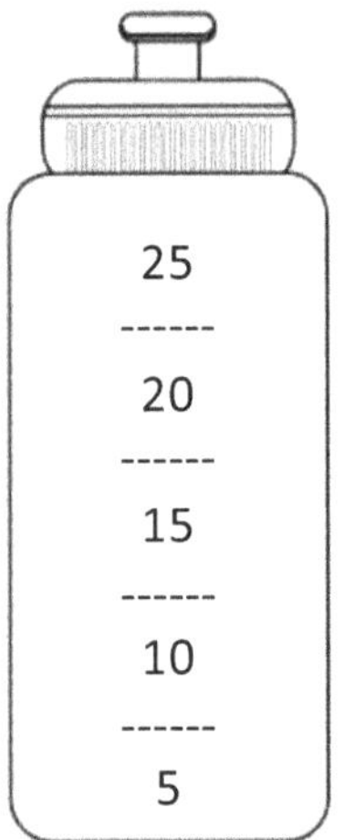

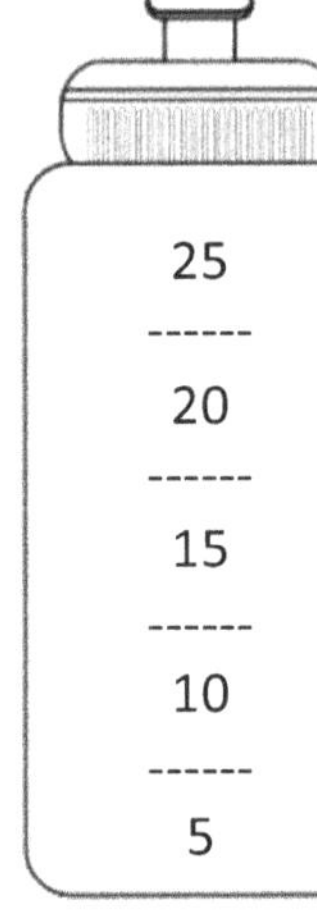

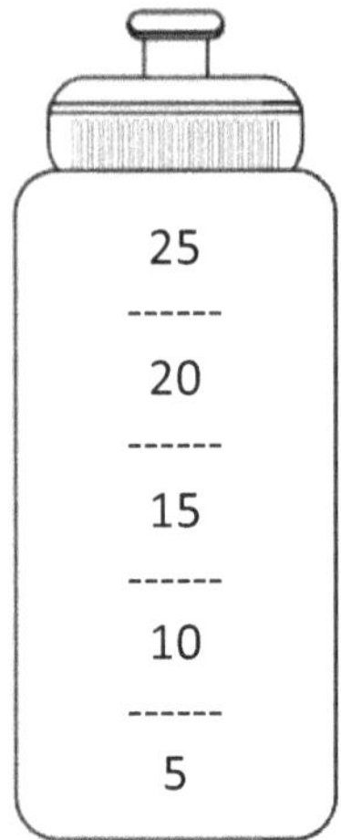

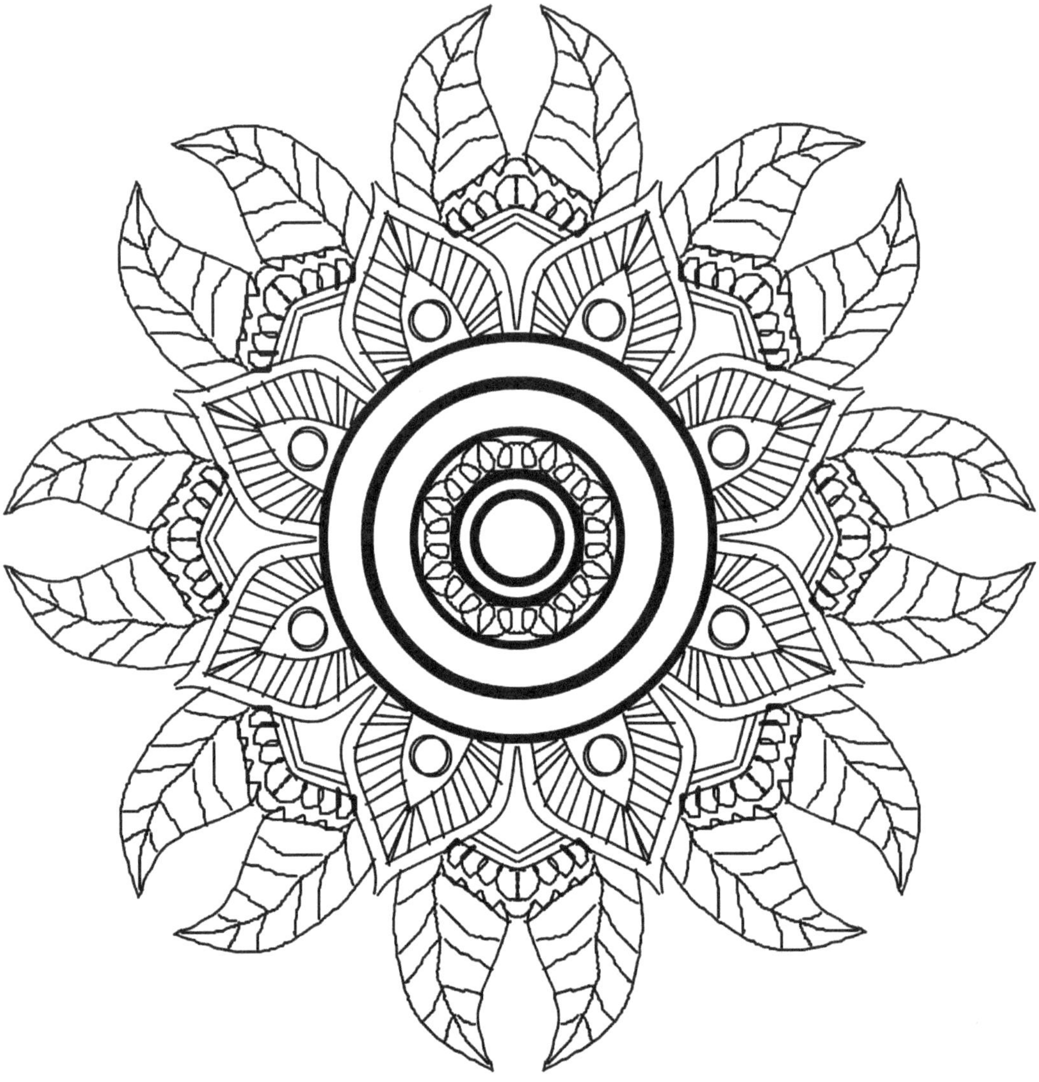

NOW WHAT?

www.ingramcontent.com/pod-product-compliance
Lightning Source LLC
Chambersburg PA
CBHW081612250726
48657CB00009B/2550